THE
ART
OF
HEALTH

THE
ART
OF
HEALTH

MICHAEL CARSON

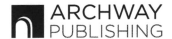

ARCHWAY
PUBLISHING

This book is a work of non-fiction. Unless otherwise noted, the author and the publisher make no explicit guarantees as to the accuracy of the information contained in this book and in some cases, names of people and places have been altered to protect their privacy.

Archway Publishing books may be ordered through booksellers or by contacting:

Archway Publishing
1663 Liberty Drive
Bloomington, IN 47403
www.archwaypublishing.com
844-669-3957

Because of the dynamic nature of the Internet, any web addresses or links contained in this book may have changed since publication and may no longer be valid. The views expressed in this work are solely those of the author and do not necessarily reflect the views of the publisher, and the publisher hereby disclaims any responsibility for them.

Any people depicted in stock imagery provided by Getty Images are models, and such images are being used for illustrative purposes only. Certain stock imagery © Getty Images.

Introduction image painted by Michael Carson
Cover Photograph by Gabriel Erwin

ISBN: 978-1-6657-2342-8 (sc)
ISBN: 978-1-6657-2340-4 (hc)
ISBN: 978-1-6657-2341-1 (e)

Library of Congress Control Number: 2022908455

Print information available on the last page.

Archway Publishing rev. date: 06/27/2022

To my mother, Janice, to the memory of my father, Richard, and to my amazing sister, Candace.

CONTENTS

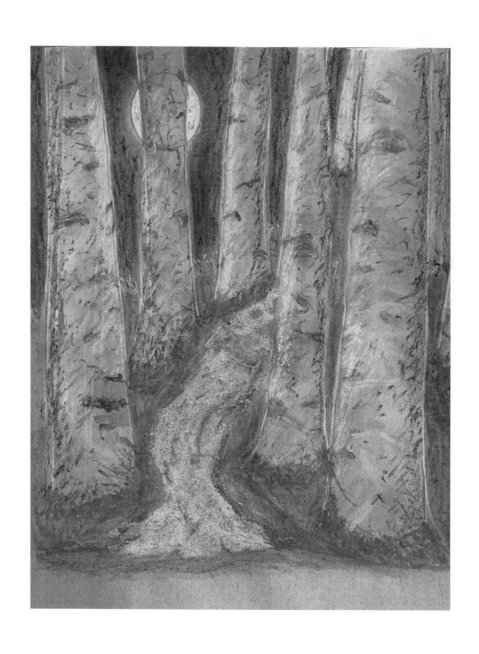

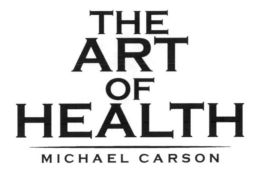

THE
ART
OF
HEALTH

MICHAEL CARSON

"To laugh often and love much; to win the respect of intelligent persons and the affection of children; to earn the approbation of honest critics and endure the betrayal of false friends; to appreciate beauty. "To find the best in others; to give one's self; to leave the world a bit better, whether by a healthy child, a garden patch or a redeemed social condition; to have played and laughed with enthusiasm and sung with exaltation; to know even one life has breathed easier because you have lived—this is to have succeeded."

—Ralph Waldo Emerson

INTRODUCTION

Health is my friend and ally, a friend I never take for granted, and one to whom I give my ultimate respect. Maintaining my health has been an ongoing journey, an evolution that has become second nature the more I understand and embrace it.

My journey started earlier than expected. I was born six weeks premature, mostly due to mine and my mother's Rh blood factors did not match. My mother's blood was making antibodies attacking my red blood cells, and this needed to be stopped or my life would end at the very beginning. Luckily, Dr. Ounatis, a visiting obstetrician from Africa, diagnosed and solved the emergency quickly.

My blood needed to be removed and replaced with Rh-factor compatible blood. Dramatic indeed, but relatively simple to correct. A heartfelt thank you to the generous person who donated blood that week back in September of 1967 when I truly needed it.

After my transfusion, there was a quick medical procedure to remove some benign abnormal growths on my head, followed by seven weeks in an incubator to build strength and become a lighter shade of purple before being allowed to go home with my parents.

At the time, there was worry that I might have future health complications due to my early birth. Nevertheless, I was an energetic, athletic child who regularly jumped over objects rather than walked around them.

While I was still in diapers, I would take any opportunity of an open door to sprint up the sidewalk and sprint right back. No escape attempt was occurring, just the desire to run. I apologize, Mom, and I thank you for not tethering me with a leash during that challenging time.

When I was six years old, Gary, a close family friend, took care of me and my sister Candace while my parents went on a needed vacation. Gary was very fit, a successful amateur bodybuilder, and the first health enthusiast I ever met.

He brought issues of *Iron Man* magazine, a pioneering workout magazine that featured golden-era bodybuilder legends Arnold Schwarzenegger, Frank Zane, Lou Ferrigno, and many others, describing their workouts and sharing their secrets for success.

The men were like superheroes to me, and I wanted to be just like them. Gary gave me the magazines to keep; I treasured them and read them from cover to cover more times than I can remember.

Soon after, at just seven years old, I started to do push-ups regularly. They were fun, and I was good at them. Push-ups shortly evolved into handstands, and by age ten, handstand push-ups. It all seemed normal to me, and thank you, Mom; a child walking on his hands throughout the house was surely nerve-racking, yet you never discouraged me. I love you for that.

At age eleven, my parents gave me a dumbbell set with an adjustable bench, and my fitness laboratory started to take form. I began creating full-body workouts, always listening to music while I exercised. The combination gave me tremendous energy and continues to. Exercise and music have kept me grounded throughout my life, no matter the circumstance.

My actual personal health epiphany happened during my last day at Pioneer Day Camp in the summer of 1979. Each year the camp held an end-of-camp Olympic-themed competition with running, swimming, climbing, throwing, table tennis, tetherball, and other sports.

I won some events in previous years, but I placed first in nine of the ten events that year and second place in the remaining one. I was amazed, and it seemed the other campers and staff were as well.

On the ride home, I was sitting with the ten medals in my hands, the song "Afternoon Delight" by the Starland Vocal Band playing on the radio. I was watching the trees fly by out the window, and felt the warm summer air hitting my face. I had never felt this good before; it was remarkable, almost spiritual, and I didn't want it to fade.

It wasn't solely about winning; it was also about how I felt physically in control of my body while accomplishing those wins. I decided from that moment on I would never let my health or energy fade.

That same month I was gifted Arnold Schwarzenegger's book *The Education of a Bodybuilder* from my godparents, Gail and Larry. Gail was Gary the bodybuilder's sister, and she knew I was interested in exercise. The book was perfectly timed; I now had the tools and knowledge I needed—or so I thought.

I was still young, pre-puberty, and not yet focused on the nutritional component of health, just performance and appearance. I hadn't made the vital connection that food is fuel; adapting that critical component into my health journey was still years away.

After high school, I studied kinesiology, anatomy, and nutrition at the University of California Los Angeles (UCLA). Stuart Rugg was my inspirational anatomy and nutrition professor, a competitive triathlete, and a brilliant communicator who would instill in me the power of food as fuel for performance and recovery from a competitive athletic perspective. Rugg was passionate and intense, and I was 100 percent on board.

Nutrition was the final piece of the health and longevity puzzle I needed. Improving and balancing my nutrition has provided me with the most significant health and recovery benefits over any other component of my health.

While studying at UCLA, to pay the bills, I began work as a production coordinator for the surfwear company BodyGlove.

My boss, a weekend athlete, noticed I was in decent shape and asked if I would be willing to train him before work a few days a week. Train my boss? This was unexpected and was the unofficial beginning of my fitness career. It was time to assume the role of instructor and coach, and I was ready.

We trained for two years until he moved for a better job, and I officially decided to pursue fitness as my career. I responded to a help wanted ad in the UCLA *Daily Bruin* and landed a job as the front desk attendant at Roebics, an exclusive fitness studio in Century City owned by my dear friend, fitness and finance guru Joey Luna.

When not working at the front desk, I took every class allowed. Joey noticed my passion and proficiency and graciously invited me to join him to learn this new fitness method called Step Reebok, with classes launching at Roebics. Step Reebok was the catalyst for my entire group exercise career, and Joey showed me the possibility.

Music had always been a part of my workouts, but Joey taught me to recognize the four and eight count in songs, understand the significance of tempo and beats per minute, and understand movement transitions. It was like giving art supplies to an eager painter;

I could create physical art while improving health and performance. Fitness was now paying my bills and also evolving into entertainment. It was an exciting time.

I developed sixty-minute routines incorporating movement patterns from sports, dance, and martial arts, and developed movement sequences for creating the most capable physiques possible, always in conjunction with fantastic music.

My workouts were intense and always fun. Members of the studio began asking me to train them privately. Private training was a bit more lucrative and easier on the body than group exercise was, and I could continue to do both.

In time, with Joey's blessing, I departed from Roebics to work at Mezzeplex, a state-of-the-art luxury health facility partly owned by fitness guru Kathy Smith. I started three hours a week as a towel boy, talked my way into being a substitute group exercise instructor within a month, and was established as the club's Group Exercise and Private Training Director by month five. I had indeed found my niche.

Soon Kathy Smith requested me as her trainer, video consultant, backup performer, and eventually a featured presenter. These opportunities led me to choreograph and appear as a featured health expert in countless television, infomercial, magazine, and fitness video productions.

Mezzeplex was also the spot to meet like-minded athletes.

A member asked if I wanted to run the Los Angeles Marathon with him in place of his injured friend. It was just seventeen hours before the race, and I had never run more than a 10k, but I eagerly accepted.

The marathon was the freest four hours and three minutes I had ever felt in my life; I even taught the group exercise classes scheduled for the next day. My physical conditioning was paying off.

Certain places and times in life define our path; Mezzeplex was that type of place and time. Working there provided me with the opportunities I needed to construct my career, compete in 300-mile adventure races, and design products and programming for myself, Reebok, The Spectrum Clubs, Equinox Fitness, the YMCA, and work on countless fitness videos and television projects. My programming continues to be utilized and prescribed by doctors, therapists, and psychologists worldwide.

My most crucial health innovation is highlighted in Chapters 9 and 10. It explains the method for consistently losing unwanted fat and maintaining metabolic health with merely ninety seconds of movement correctly timed before meals.

I always practiced what I preach; every strategy I share I have experienced personally and with clientele for many years.

This book has the potential to improve many aspects of your life, no matter your current state of health.

CHAPTER 1

HEALTH IS IN OUR OWN HANDS

If you are not your own doctor, you are a fool.

—Hippocrates

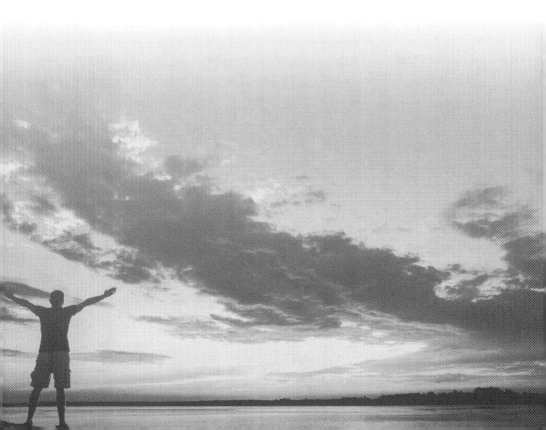

PRIORITIES

Before takeoff, the flight attendant explains that, in case of a sudden loss in cabin pressure, a mask will be deployed with oxygen to assist your breathing, but if traveling with a small child or person needing assistance, you must secure your mask first before assisting others.

It is essential to treat your health the same way. Your health impacts the quality of your life and those around you. Health must be about you first, then those around you, and then your community.

NIP, TUCK, AND ROLL

Many try, but the reality is that you will not find safe, sustainable health solutions from the use of pharmaceuticals, extreme workouts, low-calorie, restrictive diets, or continuous elective cosmetic procedures.

The most successful approach to improved personal health continues to be sustainability and longevity.

The universal agreement is that improved hydration, consuming healthy foods, and being physically active will enhance the health of anyone, including you. Physical ailments and emotional barriers will often disappear when we are healthy in body and mind, making elective procedures no longer wanted or worth the health risk.

WARNING!

The medical and pharmaceutical industries need to continually diagnose us as sick and prescribe medications and treatments for continued success. Looking for good health from an industry that profits mainly if we're sick is genuinely not a sound decision.

You would never dine at the Big Pharma restaurant if the server said to you, "The chef would like to remind you that your meal may cause severe nausea, headaches, bowel bleeding, thoughts of suicide, and fits of rage, and with the poached salmon, there's a chance of sudden death. In addition, the chef, restaurant, and I do not accept any liability or responsibility for any adverse side effects experienced from consuming your meal. So would you like to start with the Caesar salad or lobster bisque? If the bisque, someone will need to drive you home. Or wait four hours before you drive or operate heavy machinery."

Just imagine what the dessert could do to you.

Every pharmaceutical advertisement and medicine label includes a similarly long list of unpleasant side effects produced by taking those medications. Logic should steer you in the opposite direction.

There are two doctors that men and women should visit regularly, The Dentist and the Dermatologist. We discuss the importance they have in your overall health in Chapter 2.

GOOD HEALTH IMPROVES
ALL OUTCOMES

Any surgical procedure can have complications, weaken the immune system, and require additional medications that can compromise your health. When in a good state of health, healing after any procedure—from dental work to child-birth—will be faster, smoother, and with fewer complications.

PERFECTION IS NO GOAL;
CONSISTENCY GIVES YOU CONTROL

Perfection as the goal for health is not possible and is often used as an excuse to skip the steps needed to improve health or stop trying entirely.

Quickly check out these definitions from Merriam-Webster. Which is realistic, and which is improbable?

Per·fect
/ˈpər-fikt/
adjective
free from any flaw or defect in condition or quality; faultless.

Con·sis·tent
/kən-ˈsi-stənt/
adjective
acting or done in the same way over time, especially to be fair or accurate.

Being consistent gives you the best chance for success. Nobody can be perfect; however, everyone can become consistent with effort. That consistency creates lasting improvements that support continued health.

TAKE CONTROL OF YOUR DESTINY

If you are not healthy, it is your responsibility to change it. You are in complete control of your health—not doctors, trainers, therapists, or dietitians. These professionals can help, but daily, only you control your health. The power is solely yours; never take it for granted.

Health is a state of physical, mental, and social well-being, not only the absence of disease or infirmity. Remember that health must be about you first, then those around you, and then your community.

Maintaining our health is an artistic achievement, a life-long masterpiece to be appreciated, and every great work of art is a blank canvas before any paint is ever applied. Hygiene is a critical part of continued healthiness and will be the first brushstroke applied to begin your masterpiece of personal health.

CHAPTER 2

HYGIENE AND SUPPORTING HABITS

Man does not live by soap alone, and hygiene, or even health, is not much good unless you can take a healthy view of it or, better still, feel a healthy indifference to it.

—Gilbert K. Chesterton, "On St. George Revivified"

SELF CARE
ISN'T
SELFISH

HYGIENE

1. a science of the establishment and maintenance of health.
2. conditions or practices (as of cleanliness) conducive to health.

Hygiene determines the quality of your life, is essential for overall health, and is the primary reason life expectancy today is twice that of our ancestors.

Hygienic habits produce positive health benefits for the body and the mind. Self-care and personal hygiene are opportunities to reconnect with the essence of our being and provide conscious and subconscious influences that possess immeasurable benefits to our total health.

When embraced consistently, these simple hygienic habits enrich your health and help provide a strong foundation for continued success.

YOUR SMILE

The mouth reveals much regarding the health of the body and mind. Poor oral health may lead to decay, tooth loss, gum disease, diabetes, heart disease, and stroke.

Neglecting oral hygiene will also impact self-esteem and heighten social anxieties.

Consistent dental care and corrective procedures will help minimize these health risks, avoid unnecessary expenses that poor dental and periodontal healthcare will cost, and experience less discomfort during dental visits.

Practical tools to have include

- toothbrush
- toothpaste
- interdental brush
- floss
- mouthwash/mouth rinse

BRUSHING

Brushing the teeth in the morning removes acids and bacteria that build up overnight and stimulates needed circulation in the gums and muscles of the face.

When able, brush the teeth and/or use an interdental brush or dental floss to remove food debris and bacteria between teeth and gums after meals.

Always brush your teeth before sleeping.

INTERDENTAL BRUSH

An interdental brush is an excellent tool for keeping teeth clear of food debris and stimulating circulation in the gums between brushings and before brushing and flossing.

Use an interdental brush between teeth to remove any food or debris before brushing, avoid plaque buildup, and stimulate circulation in the gums

Remember, to also brush the tongue gently, or use a tongue scraper to remove dead skin cells and bacteria to help improve breath.

FLOSSING

Floss at least once daily. Best at the end of the day before going to sleep, to help remove the plaque that will naturally build up on the teeth throughout the day.

Flossing will help prevent cavities, avoid gum disease, and lower the risk of the cardiac conditions gum disease can create.

Flossing also stimulates blood flow to the gums to help keep teeth firmly rooted in healthy, well-circulating tissue.

Use unwaxed floss when possible. The additional friction against the teeth helps to remove plaque more effectively.

Using a mouthwash or mouth rinse after brushing and flossing will help eliminate other bacteria.

VISIT YOUR DENTIST
LIKE CLOCKWORK

When it comes to oral health, the frequency of professional care can make a difference. Visit your dentist minimally two to four times a year for teeth cleanings and checkups. This frequency will be best to maintain your oral health. Although, you should consult your dentist if you experience discomfort that persists longer than seven to ten days.

THE EYES

When we blink, this forces particles and debris away from the eyes that collect around the eyes and eyelids. This debris can cause the eyes to become irritated, making them feel heavier, and may compel you to rub them, transferring additional bacteria and oils from the hands to your eyes.

Always wash your hands before cleansing your eyes. Use warm water and a gentle facial cleanser/soap. Rinse above the eyes and between the eyebrows and eyelids, avoiding the eyes themselves. You can also rinse around the eyes after washing your hands with just water to help remove debris; thoroughly dry the area afterward.

Cleanse these areas between showers when needed to refresh the eyes and revitalize you.

THE EARS

Practical tools to have include the following:

- Q-tips
- facial tissues

The ears are superb bacteria, fungus, hair, and debris collectors. Keeping the ears clean and dry will help avoid ear and hearing-related illnesses.

After showering, bathing, swimming, or washing the face, first dry the ears thoroughly with a towel or tissue, and follow by using a Q-tip or equivalent to gently remove the remaining moisture and debris from the inner ears.

Protect the ears from transferred bacterial buildup by regularly cleaning earplugs, earphones, and earbuds.

NOSE AND SINUSES

Practical tools to have are facial tissues.

While we sleep, mucus and debris build up in our noses and sinuses. Removing this buildup allows better breathing and decreases the chance of getting common colds, infections, and illnesses.

It is essential to clear the sinuses after sleeping to remove the naturally occurring congestion that builds overnight and to easily avoid illnesses that can develop from clogged sinuses. Sinus infections will not manifest when they cannot take hold.

To help initiate sinus draining, place pressure with your fingertips and tissue next to the nose and under the eyes. Keep the mouth and lips closed firmly, and gently force air through your nose into the tissue. Alternating pressure on each side of the nose will help this process.

Be patient with this process; it may take several attempts to initiate sinus-clearing; this is normal. The sinuses may continue to drain for several minutes after they begin to unclog.

As you become more active in the morning, the sinuses may continue to drain. Keep removing debris until the sinuses have cleared. You will know the sinus areas have cleared when breathing in and exhaling; you have unobstructed airflow through both sides of the nose.

Clear sinuses improve breathing and significantly reduce the chance of suffering sinus and nasal infections. Any time of day or night, if you need to breathe through your mouth to get air, it's time to drain your sinuses.

Brushing the teeth or taking a warm shower or bath can help stimulate movement in the sinuses if they are significantly clogged.

Before sleeping, clear your sinuses for optimal breathing and better rest and recovery from the day.

Sinus infections are one of the top conditions for which antibiotics are prescribed. However, studies show that antibiotics only have an efficacy of 2 to 10 percent in healing these types of infections.

Avoid antibiotics whenever possible to prevent reducing their effectiveness. Antibiotics are miraculous medicinal tools that should only be relied upon when necessary to ensure their usefulness in the body.

SHOWER'S POWER

Morning showers remove sweat, bacteria, and dead skin cells built up on the skin through the night. They elevate heart rate, rapidly direct blood flow throughout the body, and are an organic wake-up call for your nervous system.

Showering before bed removes the oils, dead skin cells, bacteria, funguses, and acids that have naturally accumulated on your skin throughout the day and will help you to rest and recover better.

Hot showers dry the skin; apply lotion or essential oils to the body and face after hot showers to soothe and help protect the skin.

During the winter months and in dryer climates, use therapeutic lotions and oils between showers to help relieve the excessive itching and pain that dry skin can create and for improving the skin's appearance.

When you exercise, your pores will open, and the sweat and bacteria that build up can cause skin irritation and acne.

After exercising or sweating excessively, quickly rinse off or take a complete shower.

SKIN EXFOLIATION

Practical tools to have:

1. loofah
2. long handle exfoliating brush to reach the back
3. moisturizing lotion or essential oils

We shed approximately 30,000 to 40,000 dead cells from our skin every minute. The body naturally creates an entirely new skin for itself roughly every forty days.

Regular exfoliation clarifies the skin, improves dermal circulation, and assists lymphatic drainage to help remove waste and toxins.

Exfoliate the entire body once or twice monthly to enhance your skin's overall health and appearance. Always moisturize your skin after exfoliating to protect and hydrate the newly exposed dermal layer.

THE FACE AND NECK

The face and neck are traditionally the most exposed body parts to the elements. Bacteria, oils, makeup, sunblock, and environmental toxins can clog pores; and create skin irritation, irregularities, and various types of acne.

Only millimeters of physical change redefine the appearance of our nose and face. When pores are clogged, the nose appears more prominent, less defined, and the skin becomes inflamed.

A sustainable and realistic approach needs to apply to every health category, including our skin. Proper hydration, combined with excellent skincare, will remove years from the skin's appearance, safer and longer-lasting than any injection or filler-type procedures claiming to achieve the same.

Washing the face and neck daily, and deep cleansing pores weekly to help remove blackheads, bacteria, and debris will clarify, rejuvenate, and maintain the skin. Gently remove blackheads and bacteria when cleansing the skin, while being careful not to push oils and bacteria farther into the layers of the skin.

Using warm water helps open pores naturally for safely cleansing the face and neck. Always moisturize after cleansing the pores. Add sunblock, including a UVA/UVB protection of at least 30 SPF if planning to be outdoors during the daytime. Use the fingertips to massage upward and inward in a circular motion, drawing circulation to the skin and stimulating the face, neck, and forehead muscles.

Esthetician appointments every four to six weeks are also a luxurious gift of skin health that I highly recommend. The esthetician can help you understand your skin's specific needs.

VISIT THE DERMATOLOGIST

We all have damaged skin, no matter how diligent and meticulous our efforts are.

I trained outdoors for most of my career, and I was not concerned about the sun's power. That was not the correct approach; please learn from my mistake and use sunblock diligently.

Since twenty-eight years old, to date, dermatologists have removed nearly 1,000 pre-cancerous and squamous cell carcinoma sites from my body.

There is no safe way to tan. Every time we tan, we damage our skin, accelerate skin aging, and increase the risk of skin cancers.

To best understand the current state of your skin health, visit your dermatologist at least once yearly, or as needed to stay ahead of skin problems.

During the fall and winter months, the sun is less harmful; and are the best seasons for healing the skin from dermatology procedures.

If you observe abnormal skin growths or rashes that stay longer than seven to ten days, have them checked out by your dermatologist.

Scheduling your dermatologist and dentist visits in the same week or month of the year will help you keep a consistent self-care schedule.

Sunlight consists of two types of harmful rays: UVA rays and UVB rays. Overexposure to either can lead to skin cancer.

- UVA rays (or aging rays) can prematurely age your skin, causing wrinkles and age spots, and can pass through window glass.
- UVB rays (or burning rays) are the primary cause of sunburn and are blocked by window glass.

The kind of sunscreen you use depends on the area of the body to be protected.

Make sure a sunscreen offers broad-spectrum UVA and UVB protection with an SPF of 30 or higher and is water-resistant.

- Creams are best for dry skin and the face.
- Gels are suitable for hairy areas, such as the scalp and chest.

- Sticks are good to use around the eyes.
- Sprays are easy to apply to children, although it is worth mentioning that currently, the FDA regulations on testing and standardization do not pertain to spray sunscreens.
- There are also numerous sunscreens made for sensitive skin and babies. Be protected, and keep your skin healthy.

THE NAILS

Nails naturally collect and transfer bacteria, fungus, and viruses. Keeping nails trimmed helps avoid problems, like ingrown nails, and helps to prevent the spread of diseases.

Soaking your nails before trimming them will help make them softer and easier to cut.

Toenails grow at approximately half the rate of fingernails; however, they collect more bacteria and fungi than fingernails, making foot hygiene crucial for toenail health.

Keeping feet clean and dry and toenails trimmed supports the overall health of your feet.

THE FEET

Foot health, cleanliness, and consistent circulation to and from the feet are crucial for mobility and life quality.

The muscles in the feet and lower legs are responsible for the blood return to the heart. The feet endure forces far greater than the body's weight for the entirety of our lives.

Lack of stimulation to the muscles of the feet will diminish blood return to the heart, resulting in the pooling of blood in the feet and legs, creating discomfort, and swelling, and may lead to chronic health conditions.

Engaging the muscles of your feet and legs is the natural remedy to avoiding foot-related health conditions. Just five to ten minutes of movement or walking throughout the day will stimulate circulation from the feet and legs to the heart for better overall health.

No matter the body's position, any movement of the feet and legs will stimulate precious circulation to and from these areas. Performing calf raises while seated or standing, or even flexing the feet and wiggling the toes while lying down, will all employ the muscles of the feet and legs to assist blood return to the heart.

Get up and move whenever seated for thirty minutes or longer. Use the bathroom, get water or food—anything that will get the feet and legs to move for sixty to ninety seconds or more.

Even brief amounts of foot movement performed several times a day will improve your health. The more the muscles of the feet and legs are recruited, the healthier the body will become and remain.

MASSAGE FOR CIRCULATION

Massage for the feet directs additional blood flow to and from these areas. The feet have specific pressure points associated with every body part. Manipulating these spots via massage is called reflexology, a method used to relieve tension, reduce pain, and treat various illnesses throughout the body.

A trained reflexology therapist can significantly improve the blood flow to and from the feet while helping to balance blood flow and energy throughout the body.

In chapter 21, Health Technologies That Make a Difference, I share three non-invasive technologies that improve foot, leg, and overall health by stimulating circulation throughout the body.

1. Bemer therapy that improves microcapillary circulatory enhancement.
2. Red light therapy stimulates circulation and cellular strength, and replication.
3. Vibration training is used for accelerated muscular contractions to improve circulation, muscle development, and bone density.

FOOTWEAR

In general, shoes are rough on our feet, restrict circulation, and create an environment for moisture, fungus, and bacteria to collect. Whenever possible, remove your shoes for better circulation and more comfort.

As we age and gain or lose weight, our feet change in size and dimension. It is important to wear footwear that fits you correctly.

When wearing shoes too small, circulation will be restricted, causing discomfort that can lead to numerous painful foot and toe ailments.

If footwear is too big, the bones in the feet can spread unnaturally, causing blisters and calluses on the feet and toes; and possibly creating the potential for tripping and falling.

THE PODIATRIST

In my twenties, and before being fit for my first corrective orthotics, I experienced chronic foot pain and numerous ankle overuse injuries from my training. Even if footwear fits correctly, you may still suffer from foot, ankle, knee, hip, back, or neck pain induced by how your feet impact the ground.

Flat feet caused me to pronate severely, roll inward and make my foot impact distribution uneven, and break my body down from the ground up.

It didn't matter that I was in good shape. Fitness level had nothing to do with it; it was my genetics, and utilizing corrective orthotics would be crucial for me to maintain my active lifestyle.

My fifth generation of corrective orthotics allows me to walk, run, and hike without any of the pain or overuse injuries I encountered in my twenties.

If you are experiencing pain, please consult with a certified podiatrist to diagnose and correct any foot issues you may have. The diagnosis and correction are painless and vastly improve life quality.

Personal hygiene and hygienic practices develop an exceptional foundation for health to be built and maintained. Without consistent hygiene, health can become a continued struggle. Remember, not perfection, it is consistency that is most important.

CHAPTER 3
TAKE A DEEP BREATH

Single moments create miracles.

—Michael Carson

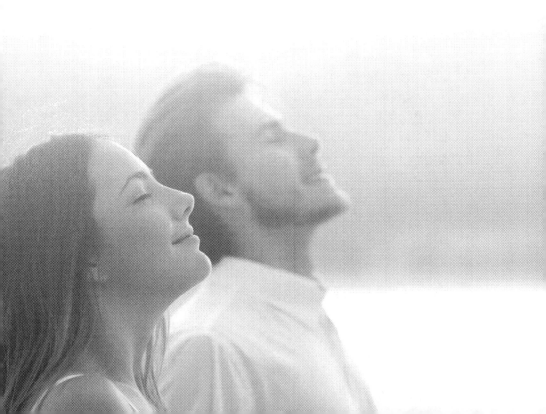

I was fourteen years old and nervous to race the fastest kids from our neighboring town in the 100-yard dash.

I started the race well and was yards ahead at the halfway point when I began to feel my body tighten up. My legs were getting heavy, and I was slowing down.

At 90 yards, one kid caught me, pulled ahead, and won by a foot and a half. I felt so defeated, but my coach, an accomplished decathlete, smiled at me as if I had won the race. I was confused.

"Michael, you know why you lost the race? You held your breath, didn't breathe, you shut down, and looked like a tomato. You only took two breaths during the entire race. You race the same kid in the 200, if you breathe, you will easily win. Can you do that?"

I was very sure I could.

I began breathing deeply a few minutes before getting into the starting blocks, focused on my breathing during the entire race, and won by almost twenty yards.

Since that day, breathing has been a significant component of my physical performance and recovery. No matter the situation, I utilize breathing to maximize my physical and mental potential.

GASSING UP

Breathing, in scientific terms, is gas exchange, the chemical and mechanical process of drawing air in through the lungs, delivering oxygen as fuel to every cell in the body, and removing deoxygenated waste and carbon dioxide from the body.

BREATH AWARENESS

Often we are only gasping for breaths, allowing stress and tension to create shallow, non-rhythmic breathing, or unconsciously holding our breath, starving all the cells in the body of the health-providing oxygen we need to survive.

In general, we do not breathe deeply enough for optimal health—only enough to survive. Improving your breathing will always promote better health and increase performance.

Be aware of your breathing when sitting at a red light, working on the computer, or performing any daily task. Take notice of your breathing, is it deep and rhythmic, or shallow and inconsistent?

BREATHING IN THE DAY

When you wake up, as soon as you remember, take four to six deep breaths.

- First breath, inhale, focusing on expanding your lower abdomen to fill the lower inferior lobes of the lungs.
- Second breath, inhale, focusing on expanding the chest and ribcage to fill the upper superior and middle lobes of the lungs.

Slowly count to four as you inhale and exhale. Repeat the pattern minimally two more times or as many as you would like.

Focused deep breathing will help you oxygenate and wake up naturally to prepare the body and mind for the day ahead. Remember, oxygen is our primary fuel source, and deep breathing raises our fuel octane level and improves health.

During stressful times, breathing can be compromised. Life-related stress and tension will physically tighten the body and can decrease your breathing when oxygen may be needed the most. Thorough deep breathing relieves stress and improves your mental clarity.

BREATHING EXERCISE

When you need to reset, or feel your best, perform the same focused inhalation cycle as the waking breaths exercise.

Take four to six deep breaths filling your lungs, alternating the focus on lower then upper mid lobes, and repeat.

Slowly count to four as you inhale and exhale. With practice, you will expand your lung capacity and easily count to six or more when inhaling and exhaling, increasing oxygen perfusion throughout the body.

Inhale and exhale solely through the nose to create the most relaxing effect. Breathing exclusively through the nose will let you know if your sinuses may need clearing.

MOUTH BREATHING

Breathing through the mouth is needed during increased exertion to help draw added oxygen into the lungs to meet the demands of the added effort.

Consistently breathing through the mouth will dehydrate the body more quickly, causing dry mouth, contributing to bad breath, and can lead to dental and periodontal issues.

Mouth breathing will also increase the likelihood of sinus clogging, create discomfort, produce headaches, and increase the chances of catching colds, influenzas, and bacterial infections.

Inhale and exhale through the nose whenever possible, or in through the nose and out through the mouth.

Limiting mouth breathing will improve your health in many ways.

A breath of health is just an inhalation away.

CHAPTER 4
HYDRATE OR DIE!

I believe caring for myself is not self-indulgent, it is self respect.

—Michael Carson

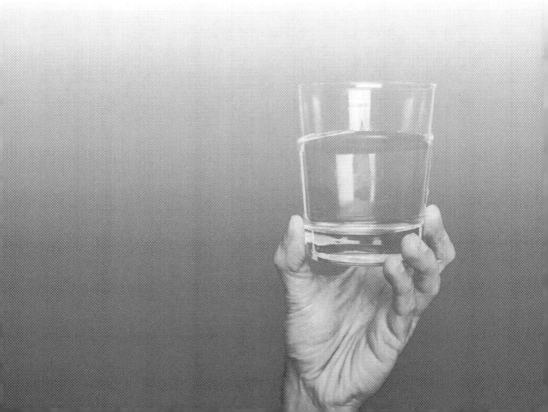

On our fifth day of the 300-mile expedition race, the Raid Gauloises in the Sultanate of Oman, my team was halfway through the 80-kilometer trekking leg in the Al Hajar mountains and had run out of water twenty-two hours earlier. We were dehydrated, in a mental fog, and moving at a snail's pace.

The race directors found us and hovered overhead in a helicopter. Yelling in French through a bullhorn, they were offering us a 1.5-liter bottle of water in trade for adding a five-hour penalty to our race time.

We were drained, with barely any energy, but we also were Team American Pride! So instead of accepting potentially life-saving water and suffering the penalty, we pulled down our pants and mooned the race directors watching us in disbelief; they hovered a few more minutes and then choppered away.

We showed them "Woo Hoo Team American Pride! We do not need your help!"…but we still had no water and were lost navigating the Omani mountains.

Maybe we made a colossal mistake. We were losing concentration and physically beginning to shut down.

We needed to get to the next checkpoint four kilometers away, where water and food were waiting.

Then we came upon a Bedouin man herding goats; I thought I was hallucinating.

We did not speak Arabic, and he didn't speak English, so we pointed to our water bottles, then our severely chapped lips. The Bedouin clearly understood what we were asking.

He turned, pointed into the distance, and began jogging away, goats in tow. We looked at each other, shrugged our shoulders, and frantically took off after him.

He was barefoot, but he and his goats were still outpacing us over the rocky terrain. He led us to a cliff edge and pointed down to a tiny pool of standing water at the bottom of a 100-foot canyon.

He nodded, smiled, and simply jogged off with his goats. One curious goat stayed behind to watch us descend into the canyon and reach the three-foot by two-foot water hole occupied by a dead snake, various unknown little creatures, and an oily substance floating on the surface. Thirsty yet? Even the goat left.

We strained the water through the cleanest socks we had into water bottles and added iodine tablets for safety.

It was the worst tasting water I had ever drank. But within minutes of drinking it, my brain and body turned right back on. It was an unforgettable experience to feel myself go from the fatigue of severe deprivation to full alertness.

I never appreciated water more; this was when I officially made water consumption a priority in life. It's hard to ignore it when you discover how vital water is to your life. I continue daily to strive for optimal hydration whenever possible to maximize my metabolic abilities and overall potential.

Water is our metabolic energy source for the over thirty trillion cells in the body. Water is responsible for regulating the nervous system, body temperature, blood pressure, digestion, elimination, lubrication for the joints, removal of cellular waste and toxins, and is a shock absorber for the brain, spinal cord, and fetus during pregnancy.

Water is crucial for every metabolic function and tissue in the body, if you are not drinking, you are not thinking.

RECOVERY TIME

While sleeping, existing bodily hydration is used to cleanse, repair, and remove cellular and bodily waste. It needs to be replenished during the day to maintain optimal health.

Hydration needs to be a daily mission. Every day you should consume water before drinking or ingesting anything else.

If you don't prioritize hydration, you will find it challenging to improve and maintain your health.

Coffee, tea, juices, wine, beer, soda, and other beverages, are not counted as water. Only H_2O counts as water.

Dehydration creates physical fatigue, mental weariness, hunger, chills, and disorientation. Even slight losses of hydration create metabolic limitations easily avoided by consuming enough water.

PREP THE METABOLISM
FOR SUCCESS

Morning hydration will determine your metabolic momentum for the entire day. Begin each day the healthy H_2O way.

1. Immediately after waking, even before using the bathroom when possible, consume your first six to ten ounce glass of water. Drink from a glass, not a bottle, to avoid swallowing additional air a bottle can create. Room temperature water is the easiest to consume.
2. After drinking the first glass of water, use the bathroom as needed. Immediately consume the second six to ten ounce glass of water after using the bathroom.
3. Consume the third six to ten ounce glass within the first hour after waking up.

For clarification:

- Drink six to ten ounces of water when waking up
- Drink a second six to ten ounces of water after using the bathroom
- Drink a third six to ten ounces of water within the first hour after waking up.

If you generally rely on coffee or other caffeine beverages for energy, I encourage you to consume water in place of those caffeinated or sugar-filled drinks for one week and enable your body to experience natural hydration energy. The effect is far healthier and the energy longer-lasting than caffeinated beverages that further dehydrate you will provide.

DAILY HYDRATION AFTER THE FIRST HOUR OF BEING AWAKE

Every waking hour, consume six to eight ounces of water.

If you miss an hour, consume two six to eight ounce glasses the following hour.

The body can only process approximately thirty to thirty-three ounces of water per hour. Only up to four to five hours of missed hydration can be replaced per hour. Be mindful of your water consumption; do not go hours without hydrating to avoid the detrimental physical and mental effects dehydration can cause.

THE DAILY H2O RULE

Every day consume approximately 75 percent of your body weight in ounces of water.

Use your body weight number and multiply that by .75.

For example: if you weigh 150 pounds, 150 x .75 = 112.5

Someone weighing 150 pounds should drink approximately 112.5 ounces of water each day, or roughly seven ounces per hour over a sixteen-hour day. Hydration also comes from the fruits and vegetables you eat, providing anywhere from 10 to 30 percent of your daily water intake.

Remember that eighteen to thirty ounces of water are consumed during the first hour you are awake, making the needed average hourly consumption only five to seven ounces of water for optimizing your health.

When adequately hydrated, the body is 75 to 80 percent water. Here are some water percentages for numerous parts of the body.

- The brain is over 80 percent
- The heart is 75 percent
- The lungs are 83 percent
- The skin is 64 percent
- The muscles and kidneys are 79 percent
- The bones are 31 percent
- Being sufficiently hydrated may increase the frequency you visit the bathroom and should be

the desired metabolic reaction. Each time you remove more waste and toxins, reduce inflammation and relieve pressure throughout the body.

If suffering from constipation, proper hydration helps to normalize elimination. Focus on daily hydration goals to naturally support mobility in that area.

During the first few days of regulating your hydration, you might use the bathroom more frequently. Your body holds on to toxins when not provided enough water. The body needs to utilize what water is present for necessary metabolic functions.

When you ingest the amount of water in access to what is required for the critical metabolic processes of the body, more removal of waste can begin. And the reason you may experience going to the bathroom more often when initially hydrating correctly.

The total health benefits of this hydrating process are well worth the additional visits to the bathroom.

Remember: if you aren't drinking, you aren't thinking.

CHAPTER 5
FOOD IS FUEL

If you think taking care of yourself is selfish, change your mind.
If you don't, you're simply ducking your responsibilities.
—Ann Richards

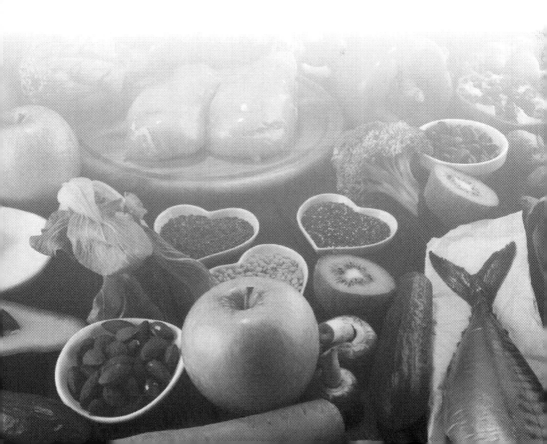

There are very few things in life you can access multiple times each day to powerfully reinforce your health and help you potentially feel your best.

Food provides you that power, the foods consumed throughout life are your body's only building blocks. They determine the state of your existing and future health.

Consuming too much of the wrong foods; or following a calorie-restrictive diet that removes carbohydrates, fats, or protein leads to metabolic imbalances, weight gain, the health risks associated with weight gain, a weakened immune system, and an increase in every health risk.

Health is best maintained by consistently eating a nutritionally balanced diet, not restricting nutrients. Correctly combining foods is chemically and physically more satiating to the body, is nutrient-rich, and is also more bioabsorbable and better utilized. Practicing balanced nutrition improves digestion, reduces inflammation throughout the body, and helps to curb cravings and overeating.

HEALTH PLAN

Eating healthily requires some simple consistent planning for maximum success. You will often make poor eating decisions when you wait until you are hungry to decide what to eat.

The more you plan meals consistently, the better your food choices. If you are not already, I encourage you to become used to preparing food and using the kitchen in general. The more control you have over your meals, the healthier you will be. You will have control of the ingredients and portion sizes and invariably spend less money when planning and preparing your meals.

THE RULE FOR EVERY MEAL

Always include protein, fat, and carbohydrates in meals and snacks.

For clarification, each meal must include:

- Protein
- Fat
- Carbohydrates

PROTEIN NEEDS A SUPPLY CHAIN

Our brain, heart, liver, and organs are primarily protein and water. Both elements are crucial for health; nevertheless, our body does not store them and they must be replaced frequently.

Protein is a macronutrient that builds and repairs muscle tissue; it is needed for digestion and the creation of infection-fighting antibodies, and it supports millions of metabolic functions that sustain life.

Animal proteins are the richest source of complete proteins. However, it does not matter if you consume animal-based, vegetarian, or vegan proteins as long as you consume enough protein for optimal metabolic function.

When you don't consume enough protein, the body becomes weak, and the immune system is compromised. The body will source needed protein from your existing body tissue for survival. This is akin to pulling a brick out of a building and continuing to remove bricks without replacing them; the building loses structural stability until it eventually breaks down. Without adequate protein in your diet, the body will react the same way.

CARNIVORE, VEGETARIAN, AND VEGAN... OH MY!

It is generally less challenging for those who eat animal protein to balance the protein, fat, and carbohydrates in meals.

Nutritionally balancing your food is crucial; vegetarian and vegan diets can traditionally be very carbohydrate-heavy.

To help you create the most nutritionally balanced meals, I encourage vegetarians and vegans to educate themselves as thoroughly as possible regarding plant-based proteins and protein-building combinations.

Here are several examples of non-meat-based protein sources for vegetarians and vegans, which animal protein lovers may also enjoy.

Non-meat complete proteins:

- Fish
- Dairy (like milk, yogurt, and cheese)
- Eggs

Plant-based complete proteins:

- Quinoa
- Soy
- Buckwheat
- Hemp
- Chia seed
- Spirulina
- Tempeh
- Amaranth

FOOD COMBINATIONS THAT PROVIDE COMPLETE PROTEIN

- Whole-grain pita bread and hummus
- Peanut butter on whole-grain toast
- Spinach salad with nut and seed toppings

- Steel-cut oatmeal with pumpkin seeds or peanut butter
- Lentil soup with a whole-grain slice of bread

SIZE IS EVERYTHING

(using animal protein amounts for reference)

Every meal, eat roughly half the size to the full size of your palm in protein. This is approximately twenty to thirty grams.

The body can only metabolically utilize up to about thirty grams of protein each meal. Consuming more becomes waste, and requires more digestive energy and hydration to pass through the digestive system.

The digestive tract must function like a smooth-rolling conveyor belt; too much protein can jam up the system and create digestion and constipation issues.

THE FIRST BITE

Whenever possible, take the first bite from the highest protein source in your meal. Consuming the first bite or two of protein stimulates digestive enzymes to break down protein for more quickly rebuilding body tissues. It also helps to keep glucose and insulin levels low post-meal, satiate hunger faster, and decrease post-meal cravings.

Beginning each meal with the carbohydrate-rich portion stimulates an unavoidable inflammatory response that can make it harder to feel full, spike insulin levels, and create post-meal cravings.

FAT WILL PROTECT YOU

Fat is our nutritional ally and slows down the absorption of carbohydrates, helps regulate blood sugar, provides sustained energy, supports cellular growth, protects the organs, provides elasticity to the skin and connective tissues, and insulates the body for warmth.

Fats are required to absorb the essential vitamins A, D, E, and K and assist in hormone production. Eliminating fats from your diet will increase inflammation; food cravings and can lead to type 2 diabetes. Eating good fats and small amounts of bad fats will not make you fat. Again, eating good fats and smaller amounts of bad fats will not lead to fat gain.

FAT GETS ONE THUMBS UP

Every meal, consume approximately the size of your thumb in good fats.

CARBOHYDRATES PACK A PUNCH

Carbohydrates are your body's primary source of energy—carbohydrates fuel the brain, kidneys, heart muscles, and central nervous system.

Fiber is also a carbohydrate and aids in digestion, promotes elimination more naturally, helps you feel full, and helps to keep cholesterol levels in check. Consume approximately 25 grams of fiber for women and 30 grams for men daily to maintain healthy elimination.

At each meal, you should consume approximately the size of your fist in healthy carbohydrates.

RULE TO FOLLOW

Every meal should contain approximately:

- 30 percent protein
- 30 percent fat
- 40 percent carbohydrates.

Adjusting to the 30/30/40 balance in your diet will help you naturally eliminate food cravings and overeating.

WHAT TO INCLUDE IN MEALS

With lunch and dinner meals, consume a small- to medium-size salad that includes ingredients like leafy greens, vegetables, fruits of all colors, nuts, seeds, herbs, sprouts, and legumes.

Salads combine concentrated energy from the earth that we absorb and utilize to enhance every aspect of our lives.

If having salad as your meal, still follow the 30/30/40 equation as a nutritional guideline. Always include a balance of protein, good fats, and healthy carbohydrates for better digestion and nutritional absorption.

HEALTH FROM FRUITS AND VEGETABLES

Salads provide the body with remarkable nutrients; here is a breakdown of some of the incredible health benefits that fruits and vegetables provide.

- Red, blue, and purple vegetables and fruits usually contain anthocyanins that help limit free radical damage to cells, and lower the risk for heart disease, stroke, cancer, macular degeneration, and memory problems.
- Red fruits and vegetables usually contain lycopene and help to reduce the risk for cancer and heart disease. They also provide potassium, vitamin A, vitamin C, and folate. They can naturally help to improve and maintain vision health and immune system strength, and reduce the risks for urinary tract infections.

- White fruits and vegetables can help lower the risk for heart disease and colorectal cancer, and are excellent sources of potassium, vitamin C, folate, niacin, and riboflavin.
- Yellow and orange fruits and vegetables with carotenoids, folate, potassium, bromium, and vitamin C will help improve immune function and lower the risk for heart disease.
- Green fruits and vegetables contain indoles, are rich in vitamin A, vitamin C, vitamin K, and folate, and will help lower the risk for many cancers.
- For salad dressing, use olive oil with a squeeze of lemon or splash of vinegar of choice; the combination will aid digestion and nutrient absorption of the salad.

As a child, I was not fond of salad, and I would only eat sliced cucumber and tomato under protest. When I finally incorporated salad into my daily diet, my digestion transformed, my endurance increased, and the quality of my life wholly improved. Now I also see the health benefits of the vegetables and fruits I choose. Knowing the benefits makes consuming them even better. I wish I hadn't waited so long.

CHAPTER 6
A LITTLE HELP FROM MY FRIENDS

The best feeling in the world is finally knowing you took a step in the right direction, a step towards the future where everything that you never thought possible is possible.

—Author Unknown

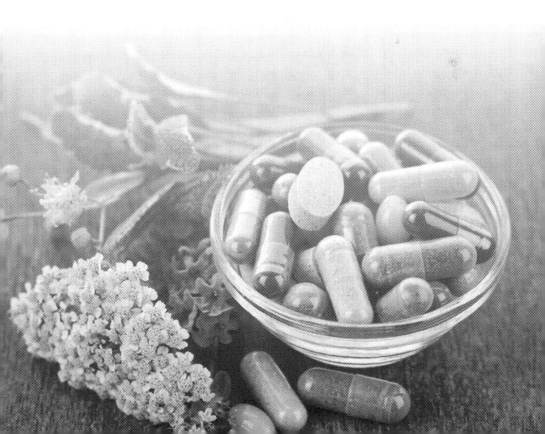

We left Port Hueneme at 6:30 a.m. in four single-man kayaks and a boat carrying a KCAL news crew, as the sun was cresting on the horizon. It was fifty-five degrees and drizzling; the ocean sounded like a gentle shower all around us as we headed toward Anacapa, a volcanic island located roughly eleven miles off the coast of California.

The plan was to paddle out to Anacapa to sharpen our caving and ocean kayaking skills. The plan quickly changed two miles off the coast when the rain shifted to hail, and the waves began cresting at four to six feet.

We couldn't see the coastline or more than twenty feet in front of us, and our kayaks were bobbing around like bathtub toys.

Anacapa Island was at least eight miles away, and my teammates were experiencing severe seasickness at the same time it hit me.

The members of the KCAL news crew were also sick, now vomiting, and told us that the storm was too rough for their boat; they wanted to turn and go back to Port Hueneme. They asked if we were ready to turn around. Honestly, we were, but we only had one weekend for this kayak training, so we needed to push forward.

They waved, turned their boat, and slowly disappeared into the mist while we struggled to remain upright in our kayaks.

One of my teammates was genuinely suffering, hunched over, and getting sick; he then lost the grip of his paddle. Because of the poor visibility, it took us several minutes to discover he was completely at the will of the turbulent ocean with no way to retrieve his paddle.

Immediately our seasickness turned into an adrenalized search and recovery mode. It took us almost ten minutes to find and retrieve the paddle. The storm continued to grow, and our exhausted teammate capsized his kayak minutes later and was now in the sixty-degree water.

We trained for this type of emergency, but in beautifully calm Toluca Lake with picture-perfect weather. Today was like *The Poseidon Adventure*.

His kayak was upside down, the paddle was gone again, and he was clinging to a rope tied to the tail end of his kayak.

That's when he told us panicking he didn't know how to swim. What the—?

We had been training for six months—plenty of time to bring it up. This rescue went from a bad day at the office to a life-and-death situation.

After several attempts with our kayaks slamming together, we finally aligned them correctly and helped our exhausted teammate onto the top of our kayaks. He was shivering uncontrollably, eyes clenched shut, and looked to be in pain as we managed to upright his kayak, find the missing paddle, and get him back into his kayak without capsizing the rest of us. His gear was saturated, and none of his food made it through the ordeal.

The storm began to calm down, but our teammate was shaking, numb, and depleted. We tied the boats together to regroup and recover. We were still about seven miles from Anacapa Island.

The seasickness and ensuing rescue drained all of us, so we could not sit idle for long. We needed immediate energy to manage the rest of the distance, and a meal wasn't an option—the ocean was still too rough, and the seasickness had not yet subsided. We needed something simple and fast. The magnesium!

A Navy SEAL advisor we worked with mentioned if he could only bring one emergency supplemental energy source on a mission, it would be magnesium—and we had some magnesium tablets.

None of us had taken magnesium before. The SEAL was not verbose; he told us to bring magnesium as an emergency if dangerously depleted but never mentioned the actual effect of taking it. Now we will find out.

About twenty minutes after ingesting the tablets with water, all of us, including our rescued teammate, were no longer seasick and felt physically and mentally ready to push on to Anacapa. Wow.

We were nowhere near our best, but the magnesium supplement took us from being four zombies bobbing in the ocean to being able to concentrate on precision paddling to Anacapa. It felt like a godsend.

Exploring the water caves of Anacapa was an incredible training experience. However, without the magnesium supplement as our rescuer, we would have been forced to return to Ventura defeated, or worse.

On our return to Port Hueneme, the ocean was like glass and perfectly still from the island to the coastline. We encountered dolphins and seals and transported several seagulls that landed on our kayaks. It was the calm after the storm.

My respect for the potency of dietary supplements and their benefits has grown significantly since that unforgettable experience. Even when following a balanced, healthy diet, some vital nutrient levels needed for the body to function at its best may still be missing.

Adding vitamin and mineral supplements will help increase healthy nutrient levels in your diet, help maximize the absorption of your food, and better regulate metabolic functions. I incorporate magnesium and numerous nutritional supplements with my lunch or dinner meals daily to maintain my health.

WHEN TO TAKE THEM

Take vitamin and mineral supplements with a meal or snack to best absorb the nutrients and avoid acid indigestion.

Do not take supplements on an empty stomach or before going to sleep, and avoid laying down for at least fifteen to twenty minutes after taking any supplements.

VITAMIN D3

1. Vitamin D3 helps the body absorb calcium, aids in preventing osteoporosis and osteomalacia, builds stronger muscles, strengthens the immune system, improves heart health, and provides anti-inflammatory effects.

Recommendation: 5,000-10,000 IUs daily.

OMEGA-3

2. Omega-3 is a crucial part of human cell membrane integrity. It improves heart health, and helps manage cholesterol, triglycerides, and blood pressure.

Recommendation: 250-500 mg of combined EPA and DHA daily.

B-COMPLEX

3. B-complex helps boost the body's defense system and keep energy levels up, both of which are crucial for maintaining a healthy immune system.

Recommendation: Take B-complex supplements that combine the full spectrum of B vitamins, including; B-1, B-2, B-3, B-5, B-6, B-12, biotin, and folic acid.

GENTLE IRON

4. Gentle iron helps produce red blood cells and avoid anemia depending on the stage of life, especially in women. The needs vary; for example, during pregnancy, the need for iron is much more than it will be after menopause.

Recommendation: 25 mg daily

VITAMIN C

5. Vitamin C is necessary for repair of all body tissues, collagen formation, iron absorption, immune system strengthening, wound healing, and cartilage, bone, and teeth maintenance.

Recommendation: 65-90 mg, and up to 2,000 mg daily

SELENIUM

6. Selenium helps regulate thyroid function; it also protects the body from oxidative stress, boosts the immune system, slows mental decline, and helps reduce the risk of heart disease.

Recommendation: 40-70 mcg daily

MAGNESIUM

7. Magnesium is the fourth most abundant mineral in the body and is necessary for many metabolic processes, including building essential proteins, like our DNA. Magnesium supplements enhance exercise performance and reduce inflammation; improve insulin resistance, protein synthesis, bone formation, energy production, and nerve function; assist with blood sugar control and electrical conduction in the heart; provide relief from migraines; and reduce blood pressure.

Recommendation: For men, 400–420 mg of magnesium per day and for women, 320–360 mg of magnesium per day.

QUERCETIN

8. Quercetin has antioxidant and anti-inflammatory effects that can help reduce swelling. They are thought to play a significant role in protecting cells from oxidative stress, killing cancer cells, controlling blood sugar, and helping prevent heart disease.

Recommendation: The most common dose is 500 mg per day, but some can take up to 1,000 mg per day. Quercetin supplements may also include bromelain or vitamin C, which may help the body absorb quercetin more effectively.

VIRUS-BEATING COMBINATION

In addition to following a nutritionally balanced diet, the daily use of zinc, vitamin C, vitamin D3, and quercetin is a safe and accessible supplemental protection against viral infections and are readily available to everyone.

If you have an existing health condition or are currently taking medications, consult your prescribing physician before taking vitamin and mineral supplements.

CHAPTER 7

NO COMFORT IN DAIRY OR ITS SEDUCTIVE CYCLE

Sometimes you have to let go of the picture of
what you thought life would be like and learn to
find joy in the story you are actually living.

—Rachel Marie Martin

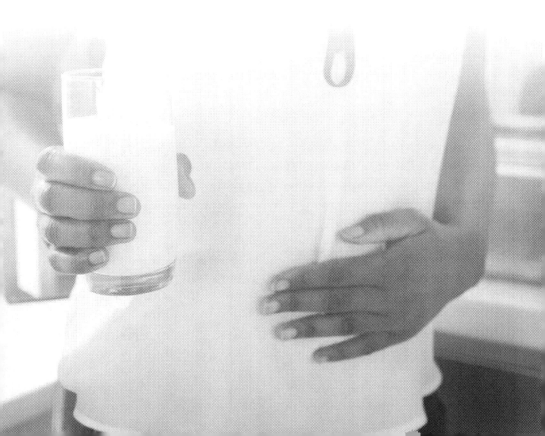

Cravings are created from feelings and emotions and compel us to take action. Comfort is the conscious and subconscious feeling created by obtaining what we craved.

The origins of our cravings and comfort demands are too vast for discussion in this book. Cravings, addictions, and habits are very closely related.

If we don't satisfy our cravings and attain even brief moments of comfort, we can feel anxious, out of control, and incomplete. This cycle becomes habitual; cravings and addictions stimulate the same dopamine rush in the brain as feeling relief, pleasure, and reduced anxiety.

Things we crave and obtain for comfort, reward, or even self-punishment provide brief subconscious, and sometimes conscious, control over our environment. We crave it and feel more in control of our world because of obtaining it.

Fulfilling our cravings and addictions can be followed by more extended periods of discomfort, emotional shame, or guilt, and may even require physical or psychological recovery. Often we forget the periods of discomfort and begin the cycle of satisfying cravings again.

That may seem like an extreme way to begin to speak about dairy. Nonetheless, the power dairy has over the population is much more of an addiction than an ally.

Cow's milk, cheeses, crèmes, and yogurts are romanticized delicacies perceived as self-reward and comfort foods. Unfortunately, the reality is dairy is a mucus-forming allergen and dangerous for the majority of the population.

No matter your lactose tolerance level, dairy consumption increases inflammation in the body, including your skin and digestive tract.

Dairy allergens induce intestinal gas and discomfort and create mild to severe digestive issues. High hormone levels in most milk, cheese, and other dairy products can also lead to numerous cancers and chronic disorders.

Baked goods generally contain less dairy in their recipes and are usually more tolerated by dairy-sensitive digestive systems. However, if even the consumption of baked goods creates digestive problems for you, you may be lactose intolerant, meaning your body does not make the enzyme lactase and cannot break down the sugars found in dairy. Those who are lactose intolerant should strictly limit or eliminate dairy from their diets.

Remember, perfection is not possible or expected; not all cravings are wrong; obtaining what we crave can give us joy and motivate us.

Cravings and comfort are a considerable part of my life, and my cravings continue to evolve with age and experience.

I crave health; I am addicted to feeling great, and I am in the habit of improving my longevity in any safe and sustainable way. Those are my primary daily dopamine sources. I love food, and I do not deny myself what I crave. But I balance those cravings in my nutritional intake to allow what I want. I never feel that I have sacrificed; I get a consistent dopamine dose while also meeting my craving to improve health.

Choosing the best dopamine delivery sources for you is essential. It determines if you satisfy cycles of cravings that reinforce our health or those that lead to physical or emotional discomfort.

CHAPTER 8
THE SMOOTHIE CHEW

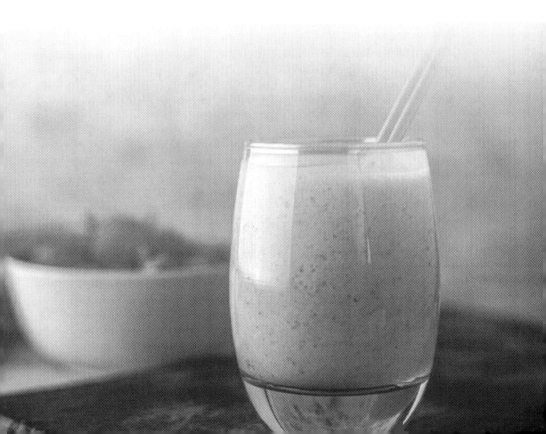

The mouth, stomach, and intestinal tract have an inseparable relationship. The mouth calls the alert and lets the stomach and intestinal tract know that nourishment and nutrients are on the way through.

Salivary enzymes released while chewing blend with the foods eaten, initiating digestion, and communicating information about the nutrients consumed to the stomach and intestinal tract to help efficiently absorb them into the bloodstream.

Without the necessary chewing that releases these essential digestive salivary enzymes, the food consumed will not be digested efficiently or absorbed thoroughly.

Smoothies and blended drinks make calorie consumption quick and straightforward. Simply chewing while consuming them—with the mouth closed, of course— will maintain ease of consumption without losing any potential benefits of their nutrients.

For clarification:

Digestion is never as complete without chewing and can lead to undesirable bodily effects, like gas and bloating. Chewing smoothies while consuming them will provide the best digestion and absorption of nutrients.

Smoothies are best absorbed in balance, and should roughly include:

- 30 percent protein
- 30 percent fat
- 40 percent carbohydrates.

PROTEIN POWDERS

Soy and whey protein powders can create uncomfortable digestive issues for much of the population. Instead, choose pea and plant-based protein powders for your smoothies to avoid any potential digestive problems and discomfort.

CHAPTER 9

MAKE YOUR METABOLISM WORK FOR YOU

Timing in life is everything.

—John Scully

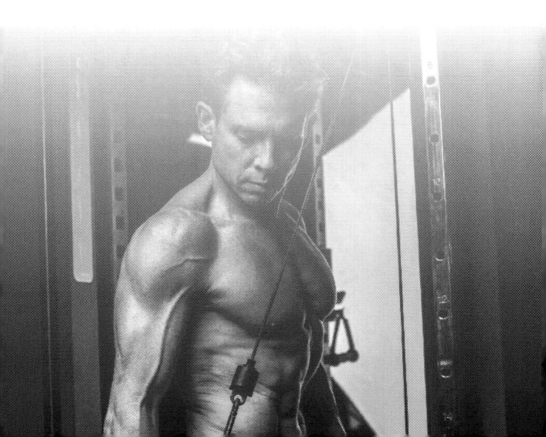

For the first half of my life, I felt I needed to push myself physically and mentally in any way possible. I wanted to test how much I could handle, how far I could run, bike, jump, lift, throw, etc. I always wanted to be physically prepared to compete or wear anybody out trying to keep up with me.

The pursuit was exhausting and extremely time-consuming. Often I would be training as much as sixty hours per week. Eating enough to sustain momentum had become a part-time job.

At one point, I hadn't taken a day off in four months. Seven days a week, I performed eight to sixteen hours of focused movement every day, including a marathon and a wilderness triathlon.

Exhausted, I realized this level of physical activity was no longer sustainable.

I was twenty-nine and nervous; if I wasn't performing all this activity, would I still be me? I had no idea; I never expected this. Admittedly I was vain and didn't want to sacrifice my appearance or my well-earned superhero-type abilities.

My passion had become an obsession no longer serving my health. I needed to figure out a solution before something catastrophic happened to me.

I spent so much time investigating and testing the latest health techniques of today and new wellness discoveries for tomorrow that I overlooked the past, our primal origins, and the ancestors responsible for our existence. The past was where I found a solution that streamlined my fitness, saving hours each week without sacrificing my aesthetics, abilities, or potential to improve.

Our ancestors didn't exercise; their existence was solely that of survival. When hungry, they hunted; and ate as soon as possible. This primal cycle enabled their survival. They would never hunt when full or satiated, only when motivated by their hunger. I needed to simulate the same metabolic response of our ancestors to achieve my goals.

No longer was it important how much training I could endure; timing the training correctly was most important. This powerful timing tool provided every health benefit I hoped to achieve.

The consistent scientific finding is that more time spent exercising does not directly equate to weight loss or increased health benefits. Exercise timed correctly allows only minutes of exertion to help achieve hours of results.

I recommend two techniques for myself and my clientele that demand the least amount of time and can provide anyone with genuinely life-changing results.

First, let's take a look at metabolism from a primal perspective.

THE HUNTER-GATHERER METABOLISM

Hunger always shows up when you need it. Hunger is your ally and provides endless opportunities to stimulate your metabolism and improve your health. Be cautioned that emotional hunger is not the same as physical hunger or dehydration, although often mistaken for hunger..

Hunger is our nervous system's signal for survival. We can also utilize hunger as a powerful tool for weight loss, reducing inflammation, muscular development, injury recovery, and mental clarity.

When our ancestors felt hungry, they had no choice but to hunt and gather to survive; while avoiding becoming food themselves.

We can still access the same primal metabolic reaction and consistently stimulate weight loss and improved health without hunting, gathering, or the fear of predators.

TWO SIMPLE PRIMAL METABOLIC TECHNIQUES

The first is a precisely timed pre-meal workout I developed that stimulates consistent fat loss and muscle development.

The second is intermittent fasting, a powerful metabolic and weight maintenance technique that only requires slight lifestyle adjustments to become second nature.

Both techniques provide safe, natural, and sustainable methods to lose fat and improve health with every meal.

Combining my pre-meal workout with intermittent fasting amplifies the metabolic results.

HAC CYCLES

The pre-meal workouts, called Hunger-Action-Consumption cycles, or HAC cycles, are ninety-second to two-minute routines. The HAC cycle stimulates the nervous system to shift into a metabolic primal hunter-gatherer mode.

You can build a HAC pre-meal workout routine with any movements you may already be comfortable performing. Include squats, lunges, stair climbing, jogging, push-ups, weighted curls, walking in place, or an endless combination of body movements and exercises. Choose between three to six moves for routines to perform for ninety seconds to two minutes for each workout.

Examples of HAC routines are also available at www. michaelcarsonfitness.com.

HOW TO PROPERLY PERFORM
A HAC ROUTINE

1. Be hungry, physically hungry; the hungrier you are, the better the metabolic reaction to the HAC routine will be.
2. Perform a routine at your current peak fitness level for a duration of ninety seconds to two minutes.
3. Begin consuming a meal or snack within fifteen minutes of completing the HAC. Eat as slowly as you like; the more you chew your food, the better the absorption.
4. If you are unable to begin a meal within fifteen minutes, repeat steps two and three to help reset the nervous system for primal metabolic mode.

HAC routines elevate the metabolism, improve digestion, and stimulate more thorough absorption of food for rebuilding the body.

No equipment is required; just enough space for you to spin with your arms extended in a circle. Take several deep breaths before beginning each HAC cycle. Keep breathing deeply throughout the routine for the most thorough metabolic effect.

Your current fitness level does not matter; pushing your body for ninety seconds to two minutes of non-stop movement completed when hungry directly before a meal is all that matters.

As your fitness level improves, so should your effort during HAC routines. The body will naturally let you know when to increase effort.

You can perform numerous HAC routines before beginning a meal or snack. Being hungry is the key. Each time you complete a HAC cycle will draw more calories from the body's stored energy sources and help build strength.

HAC cycles will also stimulate the feeling of being satiated from less food consumed. Our ancestors had limited time to ingest food and avoid predators. HAC cycles simulate this same survival digestive response. You can become full, with less food eaten and fewer calories consumed.

CURBING HUNGER WITH A HAC ROUTINE

To curb hunger between meals, perform a HAC routine, followed by immediately consuming a six to ten-ounce glass of water. The HAC routine helps curb hunger pangs by stimulating your primal metabolism for action to initiate the drawing of fuel from the body's existing energy sources.

The nervous system assumes a hunt has begun and shifts the metabolism into primal survival mode.

Our ancestors capitalized on this instinctual burst of stored energy for focused hunting to capture food to survive. We can capitalize on this hardwired metabolic reaction to burn fat, reduce inflammation, increase muscle toning, and extend life.

HAC cycles provide nervous system stimulation needed for extraordinary metabolic reactions without breaking a full sweat or even leaving your location. HAC cycles allow you to tap into the body's stored fuel sources whenever desired.

These are some of the results from a thirty-day HAC focus group with participants of varying ages and health levels.

1. The participant's lost between one to three ounces of unwanted fat every HAC cycle performed. This effect continues until the body reaches and maintains its optimal body mass.
2. The HAC cycles helped reduce inflammation by drawing the sugars that rise in the blood after meals and directing them into the muscle tissue to be used as energy, thus minimizing the insulin spike created by meals.
3. HAC cycles made it possible to spot-train the physique. HAC cycles produce a neurological adaptation, allowing participants to develop a tighter backside; and larger biceps; and sharpen coordination skills like balance and mobility. The nervous system improves those skills and movements used during the HAC routines. Our ancestors became more capable to hunt and capture

meals from this cycle. HAC routines signal the body to increase our survival abilities, and they do.

4. HAC cycles satiate hunger in a way similar to what our ancestors experienced. Eating was never leisurely or drawn-out. They needed to avoid being prey themselves. Eating was only fuel for survival; then they moved on to continue to survive. Nearly all the HAC focus group participants experienced feeling satiated sooner, with most leaving food on their plates. HAC cycles naturally encourage the consumption of fewer calories.

CHRONIC INFLAMMATION

Numerous doctors prescribe HAC cycles to their cardiac and diabetic patients as a non-medication-based solution for people who suffer from A fibrillation, type 2 diabetes, and other chronic inflammatory and digestive conditions.

If suffering from type 2 diabetes or chronic inflammatory issues, you will reduce the risks and can reduce the need for medications by performing an additional HAC routine forty-five to sixty minutes after completing meals or snacks. This pattern drastically lowers blood sugar levels and reduces bodily inflammation.

Add two to three HAC cycles before meals each day to experience better digestion and elimination, better sleep, improved muscle mass, and increased energy levels. Just three to four and a half minutes of movement timed precisely before meals and snacks.

Completing three HAC cycles a day will improve your health, and you can expect to lose an average of five to fifteen pounds of unneeded body fat every thirty days until reaching optimal body mass.

CHAPTER 10
INTERMITTENT FASTING

You will never change your life until you change something you do daily. The secret of your success is found in your daily routine.

—John C. Maxwell

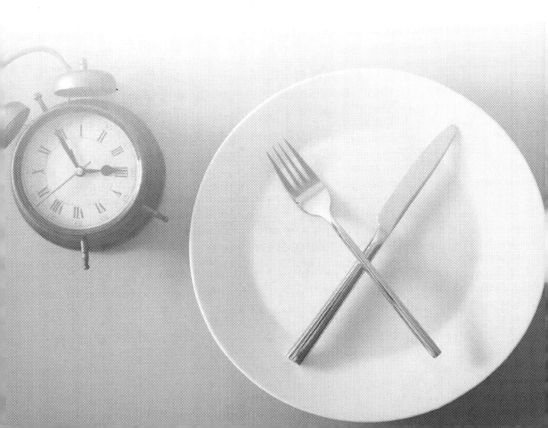

You might feel this is the most stressful time in history; our primal ancestors would probably dispute that.

Sure, they never had to merge onto the freeway during rush hour, pay a mortgage, or navigate a pandemic. Nevertheless, their days began without nourishment. Mobilizing for food and water was the only way to survive. They were always fearful of being eaten or overtaken by someone or something hungrier; or more powerful than themselves. That time in history was intense; the extreme daily stress they experienced stimulated the physiological and mental adaptations that brought us to modern times.

Their minds, muscles, immune systems, and countless physiological processes had to evolve to more significant levels for continued survival.

Intermittent fasting replicates the same metabolic process our lean and determined ancestors experienced for their daily survival. Present-day, we have the luxury to determine when our intermittent fast begins, ends; and the foods we will break our fast with.

Approximately twelve hours into fasting, glucose, and carbohydrates are no longer readily available. For maintaining metabolic homeostasis, the body shifts its fuel source from carbohydrates to stored fat. The liver then begins turning bodily fat into ketones to be released into the bloodstream for energy.. This creates a safe, natural state of metabolic ketosis. This metabolic state of ketosis remains until you break the fast. The break or breakfast can occur twelve to twenty-four hours after finishing the last meal.

Nevertheless, do not confuse a state of ketosis with a keto-based diet deficient in nutrients. Intermittent fasting naturally creates metabolic ketosis; time passing and being adequately hydrated is all that's needed.

The longer the intermittent fast, the greater the cleansing and fat sourcing effect. The window of twelve to twenty-four hours is the most beneficial for success. Intermittent fasting for longer than twenty-four hours is not advisable and can be dangerous to your health.

Intermittent fasting positively impacts chronic inflammation, improves energy, reduces fat weight, aids in regulating high blood pressure and type 2 diabetes safely, without the need for pharmaceuticals.

Nutritional intake should remain balanced when intermittent fasting for continued success; a keto diet is unbalanced and will create digestive issues. A nutritionally balanced diet with intermittent fasting is safer, healthier, more sustainable, and tastes far better than a nutrient restrictive, non-sustainable keto-based diet.

The only challenge to intermittent fasting can be the small waves of hunger occasionally experienced. These hunger pangs pass quickly and are a physical signal that the body is shifting energy sources to a ketosis fat-burning state.

Hydration is essential when performing intermittent fasting.

Follow the hydration guidelines from chapter 4 for optimal success.

For clarification:

1. Consume six to ten ounces of water when waking up
2. Consume six to ten ounces of water after using the bathroom
3. Then consume a third six to ten ounces of water within the first hour of waking up
4. Consume eight ounces of water every hour until the intermittent fast is broken.

HOW TO CORRECTLY INTERMITTENT FAST

1. Remember the exact time you finished eating your last meal. Write the time down if needed. That is your intermittent fast starting time.
2. Do not eat any food or consume any fluids besides water for minimally twelve hours from finishing your last meal. Most of this time will pass while you sleep if you start the fast in the evening.
3. Drink eight ounces of water every waking hour during your fast.

CHAPTER 11

I DO NOT HAVE ENOUGH TIME!

Tomorrow starts today.

—Michael Carson

We cannot slow, speed up, control, or bring back time. The only power we have over time is how we manage it.

I hear, "I don't have enough time" far too often. Time is precious; and how we manage our time makes powerful impacts on our health.

I do not expect people to dedicate most of their time to managing their health. But any time set aside will be beneficial and will build on itself while reducing the time needed to maintain health in the future and is vital to avoid a complete physical restoration.

I used average times to create this example, I kept the equations very simple. If you have a calculator or pen and pad, write down your hourly totals for the activities tallied to see if there are hours you may be overlooking in your week.

THE BREAKDOWN

There are 168 hours a week;

- Add an average of 9 hours a day for sleep, total-ing 63 hours a week, which leaves 105 hours left.
- Add 10 hours a day for work, seven days a week, for seventy hours total, leaving 35 hours available.
- One meal is presumably eaten during a 10-hour workday; for two additional meals, let's add 2.5 hours of food prep and eating time totaling 17.5 hours weekly, leaving 17.5 hours left.

- Estimating two hours a day of additional personal or family time, or television, computer, shopping, or laundry time, adding a total of 14 hours weekly, leaving 3.5 hours left in the week.

Even moving non-stop and getting complete rest, approximately 3.5 hours can be available every week to improve health.

Thirty minutes a day to improve health, and increase energy to help you manage the remaining 164.5 hours of the week.

Bonus:

- If you sleep merely eight hours each night instead of nine, you open up seven more hours each week making 10.5 hours available for health.
- If you work only six 10-hour workdays instead of seven full days a week, you can add ten more hours, for 20.5 hours available, almost a whole day to invest in your health each week. Work only five days? Over 30 hours reveals itself as available.

Time for health is available if we make it; any time you spend building a stronger you; is time well spent.

CHAPTER 12
THE WORKOUT

Physical fitness is not only one of the most
important keys to a healthy body, it is the basis of
dynamic and creative intellectual activity.

—John F. Kennedy

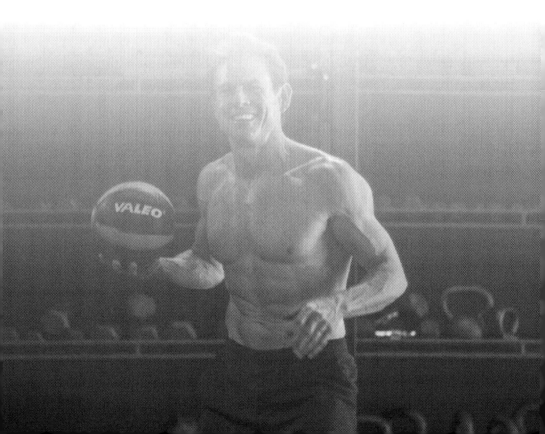

Typically the first few questions I get from a new client include these: Why do I need to exercise? What types of exercise should I do? How much do I need to do? How often should I exercise? How intense does it have to be?

They can be overwhelmed; I do not want that to be you.

Follow the same rule for exercise as you do for food: it's all about balance. The goal for workouts is to combine weight resistance training, flexibility, coordination, and balance. The whole body needs to move for everything to improve. I feel fortunate that I embraced movement and athleticism from a very young age, and it gave me an early appreciation for my health. Since I was a pre-teen, I have exercised consistently, no matter my life circumstances.

Building foundational strength and physical balance is the goal. Workouts designed to produce specific desired physical qualities are also very desirable and achievable.

Health can begin anywhere. 90 percent of my workouts occur outside of the gym, mostly in my home and outdoors.

Working out is a powerful healing tool. Even after being hit by a car with broken bones; or injured in a mountain biking crash, as soon as possible, often the same or the next day, I work the fully functional body parts to create natural growth hormones to stimulate faster healing.

THERE IS NO PLACE LIKE HOME

Never let proximity from a gym be the reason to skip exercise; the solution is much closer than you think.

Dorothy from 'The Wizard of Oz' was correct: there is no place like home, especially for improving health.

Convenience equals consistency, and we spend most of our time at home. A gym membership is a great option but always requires prepping, packing, traveling to and from the gym, and unnecessary obstacles and excuses to avoid exercise.

Gyms are perfect for social interaction, mental stimulation, and access to equipment we may not be able to afford or have space for in our homes

My health and fitness career may not have begun without the presence of gyms. However, I exercised outdoors and in my home long before any gym membership or fitness career. Most of my workouts are nowhere near a gym.

Exercising at home is efficient: it minimizes excuses to avoid workouts and is always open. The only requirement is a small space and minimal fitness tools needed to achieve consistent, completely balanced workout routines.

WEIGHT RESISTANCE TRAINING

Weight resistance training stimulates the release of natural growth hormones and endorphins, reduces cortisol levels, and helps to improve muscle strength and bone density.

Before beginning workouts, warming up the body increases blood flow and helps gently loosen up the joints, connective tissues, and muscles. When warming up, include rotational movements from the hips and waist, including squats, calf raises, walking, or marching in place to increase blood flow to the lower back, hips, knees, ankles, and feet.

THE EQUATION

You will be alternating exercises from the lower body to the upper body, then to the core, and repeat. Your workouts can also start from the upper body to the lower body and the core. Or you may begin the sequence with the core.

The redirection of blood flow this pattern develops throughout the body is the key to success.

Stimulating continued redirected blood flow during workouts improves endurance, circulation, heart strength, and stroke volume.

Blood flow redirection also burns more calories and reduces soreness by minimizing blood pooling in the muscles that weight resistance training can create. It also helps prevent overuse injuries from performing repetitive weight resistance movements.

SAMPLE 30–45-MINUTE WEIGHT RESISTANCE WORKOUT

1. Warm-up: 5–7 minutes
2. Leg or glute exercise
3. Back exercise
4. Chest exercise
5. Core/ab exercise
6. Leg exercise
7. Back exercise
8. Chest exercise
9. Gluteus exercise
10. Core/Abs exercise
11. Leg exercise
12. Shoulder exercise
13. Bicep exercise
14. Triceps exercise
15. Core/Abs exercise
16. Back exercise
17. Tricep exercise
18. Bicep exercise
19. Leg or glute exercise
20. Core/Abs exercise
21. Gentle stretch

This method keeps the heart rate up naturally during a workout and makes cardio or cardiovascular-specific exercise unnecessary. Just one workout provides the benefits of several when performed correctly.

CHAPTER 13
REST AND RECOVERY

I believe that the greatest gift you can give your
family and the world is a healthy you.

—Joyce Meyer

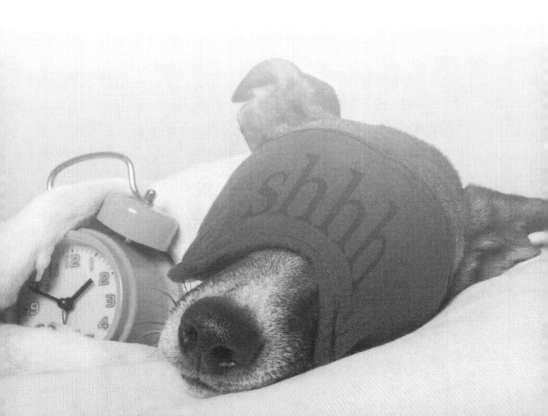

We were preparing for The Raid Gauloises, a 300 mile team expedition race set in the Sultanate of Oman. The race involved seven to nine days of navigating twenty-four checkpoints over diverse terrain on foot, on horseback, by canyoneering, mountain climbing, ocean kayaking, and a desert camel trek as the final leg.

As Team American Pride, we were the first Americans to attempt this European-dominated race, and we intended to win.

To win the race, we would need to push hard; and stay awake. If teams slept or rested, they likely would be passed by the teams that would keep pushing through.

Our team hired a licensed psychologist who had a solution for eliminating the need for extended sleep. We would get training to go from fully awake to a REM sleep state and back to fully alert in 30 minutes, which would equal eight hours of complete rest. And the doctor's accelerated REM process appeared to work lying on the floor in the controlled environment of his plush Beverly Hills home office. Now we could initiate super sleep; the other teams were in serious trouble.

Forty hours into the race, we had made it through the 36-kilometer horse ride and run, eight hours of canyoneering through frigid waters, and were part-way through the various peaks in the Hajar Mountains. It was 3:00 a.m.; we were dead tired and needed to stop for a break, and it was time to unleash our secret super sleep weapon.

We were lying on the ground at 8,000 feet of elevation, still wearing our boots, wrapped in space blankets for warmth, and ready to give super sleep a test drive.

We set our alarms for thirty minutes. The four of us lay there staring at the star-filled sky, exhausted and shivering. One teammate was mumbling constellation names as if playing a word search. One was out cold, headlamp still on, mouth wide open, snoring loudly and releasing gas from the other end like a bagpipe. The other three of us were in a daze but awake.

When the alarm went off at thirty minutes, it felt like a hammer hit my head. As we started onward through the darkness in the mountains, we all agreed that the super sleep method was closer to super stupid. We had worn ourselves out, and the strategy was no success.

A French team won the race in under seven days, swiftly navigating through the night using only the stars to navigate. They greatly outclassed us. I always wondered how much they slept?

The Raid Gauloises wasn't the only time I overlooked the importance of sleep and recovery for maintaining my health.

I burned the candle at both ends for work and training for years without an end in sight.

I was a bit intense about work; if offered, I would accept clients; to teach classes, participate in a competition, or any physical challenge, partly in worry that offers would stop if I were to say no. I felt blessed to be active and never took that for granted. But finally, it was breaking me down. Whether I wanted to accept it, I was doing too much.

Recovery and resting took time, and I considered it akin to sitting idle and failing. I did not have a healthy view of rest or sleeping at the time; my feelings have changed significantly.

I added two days of rest a week, spread three days apart. Within weeks, I was lifting slightly heavier weights, running a bit stronger, recovering quicker, and performing better in every category of my workouts.

What the hell had I been doing to myself the past few years?

Taking the time to rest also improved my physique; I looked more defined but exercised less. Overtraining had been causing my muscles to retain fluids, was irritating my joints, and continually stressing the connective tissues. The realization I had been diminishing my physique and hurting myself by overtraining changed my approach to exercise and health from that time forward.

Exercise only stimulates the changes we are hoping to achieve; without rest and recovery, none of those changes get the opportunity to fully materialize. The metabolic magic happens during recovery, when the physical changes, performance improvements, and adaptations occur.

Sleep is when the body metabolically repairs and rebuilds tissue; the only time the brain has the opportunity to cleanse itself and prepare for the next day. Without the proper rest, we become diminished versions of ourselves; and begin to mentally and physically malfunction and break down.

Consistent rest will increase your energy, improve concentration, lower inflammation throughout the body, help develop a robust immune system, and naturally elevate your mood state and hormone levels.

For athletes, rest is crucial for performance, stamina, mental focus, coordination, endurance, and avoiding injuries. Sleep recovery is truly the most powerful healing tool we have.

HIT THE SACK

Get seven to eight hours of sleep whenever possible. Athletes, and highly active people, may need upwards of nine to ten hours for the required amount of rest and recovery.

Twenty to thirty-minute naps during the day are perfect for a recharge, but keep them under an hour. Napping longer than an hour, or after 3:00 p.m. can make sleeping more difficult that evening.

OVERSLEEPING

Too much rest can be detrimental to your health; and can also be a possible sign of depression, malnutrition, or illness.

Oversleeping pools the blood, increases stiffness in the body, and increases the risk of numerous chronic ailments.

If you routinely sleep more than nine hours a night and do not feel rested with less sleep, it may be impacting your health and worth taking a closer look at what may be the cause.

Sleeping in late on the weekends is not a big issue, but it can throw off your circadian rhythm, making falling asleep more difficult when returning to the workweek.

I lost years of rest I will never get back. Now I do my best to sleep whenever possible. Sleep is also an opportunity to create your future reality, which I will share more about in chapter 22, explaining the relationship between the conscious and subconscious.

CHAPTER 14

WHICH MOMENTUM DO YOU CREATE?

The best day of your life is the one on which you decide
your life is your own. No apologies or excuses. No one
to lean on, rely on, or blame. The gift is yours—it is an
amazing journey—and you alone are responsible for the
quality of it. This is the day your life really begins.

—Bob Moawad

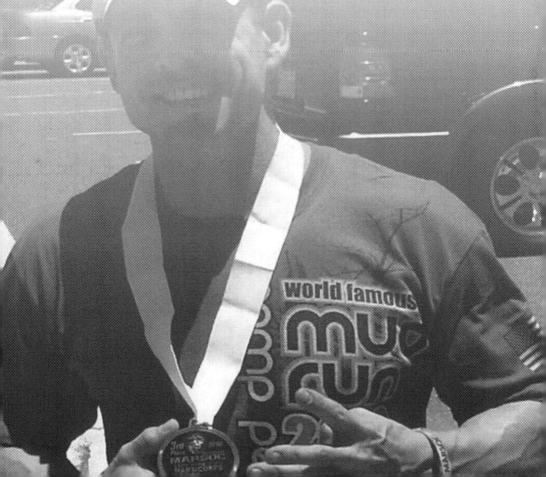

It was 7:45 a.m. and perfect San Diego weather as I began wiggling my way slowly through the thousands of participants to position myself as close as to the start line of the Camp Pendleton Marine Corps 10k mud run as possible.

Generally, races make me a bit nervous, but this was a unique situation; in this race, I wasn't running as myself. I'll explain. The Thursday before the Saturday mud run, I received a call from a friend whose son had fallen ill and was unable to run. He graciously offered his son's ticket plus a ride to and from San Diego. The mud run was precisely the type of fun opportunity I kept myself in condition for. The only thing was that his son was 22 and I was 47, and I would be entered in the 19-24 category.

We figured the approximately 7,000 runners would be covered in mud the majority of the race, so who would notice?

Minutes before the race, I made it to the front start line; I had never positioned myself in a big race this way. I looked back at the pumped-up, caffeine-fueled group of warriors, bucket listers, and military personnel, and then the nerves hit me. I felt like I was in Spain at the start of the running of the bulls, and I hoped not to get trampled.

The front of the pack was where the serious runners were, the guys who did not crack a smile or have time for any rah-rah camaraderie nonsense. One such gentleman to my left sported wraparound combat glasses, a clean-shaven scalp, and an IronMan triathlete tattoo on his calf. He was hopping up and down in place and bumping me repeatedly; with his arm.

Being bumped turned my nervous feelings into adrenalized excitement. Wraparound was a big guy, probably six-foot-two, and I'm five-foot-six if practicing good posture. His "You're in my way!" vibe was just the push I needed—a little motivation to storm this course and show my 'hoppy' new friend I meant business.

I looked back at the sea of athletes and made a mental note not to see the backside of any participants if possible.

Still being bumped by hoppy Wraparound, the countdown to start began. When the gun went off, I could feel the simultaneous exhale of nearly 7000 people and the unmistakable patter of thousands of feet pounding the earth behind me like a soundwave of energy. Wraparound was right next to me, inches ahead and breathing comfortably.

I determine when to make a passing move in a race or competition based on my opponent's breathing, paying specific attention to the rhythm. The moment someone becomes just a breath out of rhythm provides me the opportunity to make a move. It's like knocking one of the balls away from a juggler while in motion; getting that rhythm back without resetting is challenging. That reset in competition is an opportunity to overtake an opponent.

As we made the left turn into the first mud hill run, the two of us were ahead of a small group by a couple of yards and the rest of the pack by a football field.

This year was my first Camp Pendleton mud run; I wasn't aware Marines were positioned with fire hoses to knock runners down as they headed up the steep mud-covered hills and over various obstacles on the course.

The first positioned Marine missed me with the fire hose as I made a lateral move just in time, but Wraparound got tagged in the face. I heard him take a huge breath and shout an extended four-letter-word filled sentence at the offending Marine.

His breathing was now out of rhythm; it was the moment to strike. He was likely in slight oxygen debt from yelling and was a few yards behind me as I crested the ridge, prepared to freight train down the backside of the hill; downhill running was my specialty.

I created an easy-to-master downhill running technique during the 90s that reduces foot strike impact. It utilizes a reverse rotation of the arms that looks unique but is very effective. It looks like you are grabbing the air and pulling back toward yourself while running downhill. The technique counters the forward running momentum, significantly diminishing foot strike impact. I haven't seen anyone else do this. I'm not sure why; it's remarkably efficient.

With my technique, I can run full speed downhill. Running with your arms moving in the traditional forward rotation increases impact, making the need to slow down to avoid going out of control.

I was not giving Wraparound time to catch his breath; that downhill was when I left him entirely. It was muddy and steep, and I was in a total reverse arm rotational sprint. I did not see him again until after the race; he did not seem to want to celebrate together. Oh well.

Now I was alone on the course, with nobody to block my attack on the remaining obstacles. The Mud Run obstacles included sand, mud, a swim through a lake, climbing wooden barriers and cargo nets, trudging through deep sand, over muddy hill trails dodging fire hoses, multiple wood walls to leap over, a mud-covered crawl under 12-inch barbed wires, and a final 50-meter sprint to the finish. It's an awesome experience.

When I made it to the finish line, there was nobody there. I asked the first person I did see what was going on. They said, "You finished. I think you were second or third place out of the guys. Congrats."

Was I, Oh my god? I had taken third place and would receive the medal at the podium.

Remember, my entrance was as a six-foot-one twenty-two-year-old. Unless the race had been supremely harsh on me, it was best someone from his family accepted the medal; to avoid any confusion. His uncle was able to accept the medal on his behalf; and explained to the coordinators that his nephew apologized he could not stay for the award ceremony.

I held the medal briefly, enjoyed the moment, and gave it to his father to give to him. It was such a fantastic experience.

If not for the healthy momentum I developed in my life, I wouldn't have the ability to accept invitations to unique opportunities and perform at the level I have. I am so grateful for every opportunity that comes my way.

Momentum determines everything in life. The body will always react to the stimulus received. If the body is not active, it will stop adapting to movement. The nervous system requires consistent signals to be sent and received to remain physically and mentally active.

Without movement, the body will atrophy, lose muscle mass and bone density, and circulation diminishes.

Physical movement stimulates muscular growth (hypertrophy), increases energy levels, circulation, stamina, and strength, and sharpens mental clarity

MOMENTUM

Have you ever skipped exercising because you felt tired or unmotivated?

Momentum is the issue and the solution; physically moving is the most challenging but necessary part of creating momentum. When the body rests too often, the desire is to stay at rest, and the body will only do what it is asked.

The key is to break the seal with a few minutes of movement to initiate the metabolic shift for motion that creates momentum.

The metabolic spark created from just a few minutes of movement provides stimulation to signal the body for action—tiny amounts of activity will help improve health and often launch into longer workouts.

BREAK THE SEAL

Set a timer for two minutes. Begin by walking or marching in place, including movements you are familiar with and able to perform in your present location, like squats, climbing stairs, push-ups, arm curls, dips, or even dancing.

Adding music to workouts, even brief ones, helps lift energy and create momentum.

After two minutes of movement, the metabolic seal has been broken. You may even feel the urge to continue. It is okay if you do not.

Consistently shift momentum and break the metabolic seal to improve your health and naturally elevate your mood state

Creating momentum in small amounts leads to more. Continued momentum enables you infinite possibilities.

CHAPTER 15
THE GERBIL MILL

Time is the most valuable thing a man can spend.

—Theophrastus

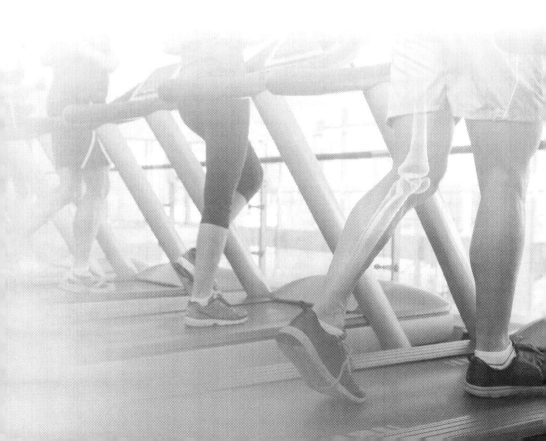

One of the distinctive characteristics of living in Los Angeles, particularly during the 90s at Mezzeplex, was the number of celebrities and pro athletes you would encounter. It was the norm to be in the locker room with an Oscar winner, Hall of Fame athlete, and grammy winner at the same time.

When I started working at Mezzeplex, part of my role was to bring clean towels to the members while they were using the cardio equipment.

Several stationary bikes were on a podium with a full view of the exercise floor.

10-time MLB All-Star Steve Garvey was on one of the bikes, pedaling vigorously. As I handed him a clean towel, he asked me. "Hey, do you happen to know that guy's name?

I looked to see it was Rock singer Billy Idol, a temporary Mezzeplex regular, there rehabilitating a broken leg from a motorcycle accident, walking with a cane, about to get on a treadmill.

"That's Billy Idol," I told him.

"Ohhh, yeah, right, why is he getting on the treadmill? That's not going to work out for him," he said knowingly.

Billy got on the treadmill, placed a foot on each side, turned it on, pressed a few buttons, put on a pair of headphones, and started jamming to what he chose to play and making a rock n roll face and air drumming while still standing on the treadmill astride.

Things looked good from where we were watching on the podium as Billy placed one foot onto the treadmill, and like a blonde spiky-haired cartoon coyote, he was immediately thrown straight into the wall behind the treadmill. Garvey said, "Whoa!, Yep, that's what I figured," and giggled as he kept on pedaling.

Billy was folded and wedged between the treadmill and the wall; as the staff rushed to his rescue. Other than some treadmill rash on his arm; and the genuine rebel yell Billy let out as he crashed, he was okay, although he did choose to use the recumbent bicycles from then on.

That type of accident could not have happened if Billy had gone for a walk instead of using a powerful treadmill. The ground would never have thrown him that way, no matter the circumstance.

By now, you understand how passionate I am about my health. I incorporate any technique or tool I have researched that can positively impact my physical or mental health.

Nonetheless, I do not and have never owned a treadmill or stationary bike.

These tools are helpful in small doses; but genuinely not the neuromuscular equivalent of the locomotion of walking, running, and outdoor cycling. These tools can get your blood pumping but do not stimulate a fraction of the neuromuscular and mental recruitment their traditional counterparts can do every second of use. Stationary bikes and treadmills; should be a substitute rather than a replacement for their more-traditional counterparts.

BIKES

There are numerous similarities between traditional bicycles and stationary bikes; they operate similarly and offer varying degrees of resistance.

Whether on or off-road, real bicycles require you to balance, steer and make millions of continuous conscious and unconscious neuromuscular adaptations and balance shifts while navigating surroundings and adjusting to weather conditions.

Stationary bikes are more straightforward; you sit, sometimes stand, and pedal. Even stationary bikes with television monitors or virtual training programs do not supply the brain and body engagement traditional biking can provide..

TREADMILLS VERSUS THE GROUND

There is a significant difference between walking on a treadmill and walking on the ground. When walking on treadmills, the belt moves, directing the feet backward, engaging fewer leg muscles, and yielding less effort than walking on the solid ground provides.

Walking on the ground requires more movement in the feet and hips and better engagement through the core and hamstrings.

Treadmills produce an unavoidable impact that creates knee stress due to the belt forcefully driving toward you as your foot strides forward.

This stress can create significant damage if improperly using a treadmill. There is a finesse to using treadmills; if you can hear the foot strikes, that is the pure impact you are asking your body to absorb.

The less impact noise while using a treadmill, the better your foot strike timing is. The farther in front of the body your foot lands on a treadmill, the more significant the impact. Aim for your feet to land more underneath your body while using a treadmill to minimize these impacts. Comparatively, walking, jogging, hiking, and running will recruit the lower leg and core muscles to generate locomotion that is more applicable to everyday life.

I will utilize stationary bikes and treadmills by incorporating them into full-body routines.

Stationary bikes and treadmills are excellent for use as a warm-up before workouts and in place of leg weight resistance exercises when doing circuit-style routines.

For leg exercises, perform thirty to sixty-second sprints on a stationary bike; or two to three minutes of walking, hiking or running at a slight incline of one to three degrees on a treadmill to minimize knee impact and increase muscular recruitment for the back of the legs and glutes.

Walk, hike, or bike outdoors whenever possible, and enhance your weight resistance workouts with stationary bikes and treadmills or when going outdoors is not an option.

CHAPTER 16

WE ALWAYS CRAWL BEFORE WE TALK OR WALK

How old would you be if you didn't know how old you are?

—Satchel Paige

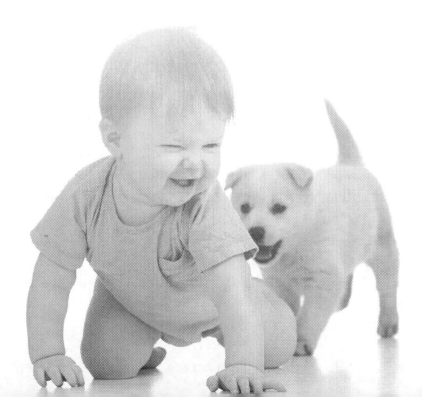

It was 8:00 a.m., and I was headed from the Tokyo airport to a hotel to freshen up and make final preparations before presenting four seminars to various Japanese athletic trainers and therapists regarding the use of vibration training. The twelve-hour flight was a bit turbulent; I only slept the first hour and felt weary from the long flight, but I had a solid plan to bring myself back to life.

During the Gulf War, travelers to the Sultanate of Oman from the United States required a sponsor who resided in Oman to visit. When traveling there to compete in the Raid Gauloises, our sponsor was Richard Simmons--not the one who first comes to mind.This one was British SAS intelligence, Major Richard Simmons, stationed in Oman to assist with U.S. and British armaments during and after the Gulf War

We flew twenty-four hours to get to Oman. Before we could unpack, shower, or eat, Major Simmons had us change directly into shorts and t-shirts and go on what turned out to be a five-mile hilly run in the Oman heat to discuss the schedule for the upcoming weeks.

Interestingly enough, both fitness guru Richard Simmons and military badass Richard Simmons choose to wear painfully tiny running shorts. SAS Richard had no shirt, socks, sunglasses, or hat.

He spoke the entire hour without pause or even a sip of water, without slowing down once. The five of us, twenty years younger, were stumbling behind him like cubs trying to keep up with papa bear. This Richard certainly was not the Sweating to the Oldies Simmons.

When we returned to base camp, Major Simmons explained when traveling to a different time zone, the fastest way to acclimate the body to local time is to walk, run, or do movements exposing yourself to the sun. The more movement done and skin exposed to the available sun, the quicker the acclimation will be.

Lying in the sun would not be the same; moving the arms and legs and body was vital for the physical and mental effects. I will forever use this valuable tool when arriving in different time zones; it has always worked for me.

Back in Tokyo, I checked into the hotel, quickly unpacked, and took a brief shower. It was 9:40 a.m.; I figured in less than thirty minutes; I could take a run around the neighborhood to acclimate myself to local time, shower again; and get to my 11:00 a.m. seminar a few minutes early. Perfect plan.

I grabbed my music; and keycard; and headed for a run downstairs wearing a modified Richard Simmons uniform: a bit longer pair of shorts, socks, and sneakers with hopes of getting as much sun exposure as possible.

I studied Japanese years ago at UCLA; this was my first trip to Japan, but I was confident it would come flooding back to me.

I walked out the hotel lobby doors and scanned the landscape. It was 60 degrees, cloudy, and resembled parts of New York City only with Japanese signage. I selected Santana on my iPod and took off for a run.

Immediately, I noticed I was the only person running. People on the crowded sidewalks were all wearing suits, even the children; were dressed formally.

I was turning heads in a way that seemed to be terrifying people. I decided it was probably best to head back to the hotel.

I turned around, jogged to the corner, and was sure I needed to take a left to get back to the hotel. I was wrong; it led me to a fish market.

I took out my hotel key card to see the address; the card only had the hotel logo, phone number, and magnetic strip.

Oh boy. Now it was 10:00 a.m., and it was beginning to drizzle.

I tried to ask several pedestrians where the hotel was, but due to the rain, people had opened their umbrellas and began covering their faces if I approached. I had been in Japan for two hours and was tormenting the community.

I asked myself what would Richard Simmons do? Not the SAS one, the other one. So I changed my tactics from polite to pleading. I went into the first business I saw, a small ceramic wear shop.

I was shirtless, dripping wet, and saw the century-old Japanese man sitting behind the counter. Standing holding out my hotel key card, I asked in my best available Japanese, "Please help me (Watashi o tasuketeku-dasai). I need to get back to my hotel (Hoteru ni modoru hitsuyō ga arimasu)."

He looked at the key card and then at me, laughed, patted my wet head, and replied, "Watashi wa anata o tasukeru," which means "I will help you."

I was relieved. The man quickly drew a precise map for me, signed it beautifully, and insisted I take a newspaper to cover my head from the rain. It was only 10:15 a.m. I would make my seminar on time; he saved my business trip.

I was no longer tired or jet-lagged; SAS Richard had given us excellent advice back in Oman. Moving your body in the sun and elements acclimates your body clock to local time quite efficiently. Although, it will do nothing for your navigational abilities.

WE CRAWL BEFORE WE TALK

Cross-crawl movements are any cross-lateral movements of the body using physical opposition, like crawling, walking, running, and swimming.

As soon as we began to crawl, those cross-crawl movement patterns stimulated infinite, complex brain and nervous system responses crucial for developing physical movement, learning language, reading, and evolving hand-to-eye coordination. Cross-crawl forges neurologic integrity and prepares the body and mind to function at their best.

Performing cross-crawl movements coordinate the brain's right and left hemispheres for electrical impulses and information to pass freely between the two, re-integrating the brain and nervous system and re-organizing the mind-body connection.

Also, every intentional cross-lateral movement, like reaching the opposite knee or foot and crossing the body's midline, coordinates the right arm and left leg, then the left arm and right leg. Or vice versa.

Initiating cross-crawl is as easy as crawling, walking, running, stair climbing, or any movements that reach across the body's midline.

Any cross-crawl activity performed even for a short time will stimulate the brain and nervous system to reset and strengthen the communication potential of the hemispheres of your brain.

You may have heard the expression—"Walk it off!"—said to us when we need to reset, refocus, and alleviate physical or emotional pain. It turns out that the simple act of walking it off does much more than take us from point A to B.

Incorporate cross-crawl activity multiple times a day to help you physically and mentally reset and function at your best.

CHAPTER 17

GET THE BAD OUT FOR GOOD THINGS TO HAPPEN

Do not let what you cannot do interfere with what you can do.

—John Wooden

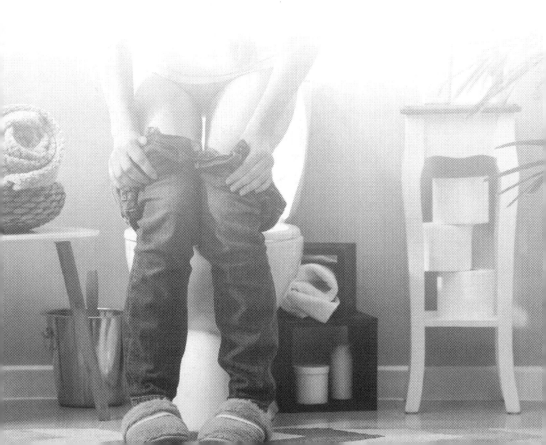

Using the bathroom is a very personal subject. In grade school, I was never comfortable defecating at school or in a public restroom until my late teens when going to college. Number one was never a problem, but two was out of the question unless I was home in the comfort of my bathroom. There is no issue when going home after school each day, but not when you are away from home for 22 days.

When I was thirteen, I went to Lost Bay wilderness camp in Ontario, Canada. We learned canoeing in authentic Native American hand-carved canoes, riflery, archery, fly fishing, dock wrestling, basic wilderness survival, and essential tasks to support a group's existence for three weeks in the woods. This year it was about learning how to eliminate outside the comfort of my home bathroom.

Lost Bay camp had a head director, but the campers ran the daily camp activities, from assembling and breaking down the activity center daily to cooking, kitchen patrol (KP) duties, and washing laundry in the lake. It was a unique camp, and there was only one bathroom: a non-flushing, wooden outhouse located directly next to the camp activity area.

I had never been able to manage a public poop in the past; I had no idea what to do besides bloat and likely be in pain.

On the fifth day, when we were returning from a day of canoeing was when I saw my opportunity. I could paddle like mad, beat the group back to the camp, and finally have privacy from the rest of the campers to take care of what was now seriously backed-up business.

There was a sign on the outhouse wall with Wile E. Coyote telling you, "Don't forget to flush!" and an arrow pointing to a bucket of sand and scoop for tossing on top of whatever business is left behind. You tend to remember special places.

My adolescent example is the opposite way to handle your personal business. I could have easily ended up in the hospital when going that length of time without elimination. Making improvements in eliminating will make a positive impact on your overall health

The act of urination and defecation removes toxins, bacteria, inflammation, and pressure from the body. Consistent elimination is a crucial component of maintaining optimal health.

BLADDER MATTERS

When you suppress the urge to urinate for extended periods, this allows bacteria and toxins to build up, which may lead to urinary tract infections and an increased risk of kidney disease.

Depending on the size of your bladder; and the volume of fluids and caffeinated drinks you consume, you should urinate approximately every ninety minutes to two hours, minimally four to ten times a day.

Whenever the urge occurs, relieve the bladder sooner rather than later for optimal metabolic health and removal of bodily waste.

Drinking six to ten ounces of water after bathroom visits will help maintain optimal hydration.

BOWEL BUSINESS

It is highly recommended and is normal to defecate daily. Some bodies go three or more times a day, some only several times a week.

Three or more days without a bowel movement is considered too long and can create complications like hemorrhoids, anal fissures, or fecal impaction. The body is continually creating waste. When "Nature calls," as they say, please go; to maintain optimal metabolic health.

If constipated, increasing hydration and consuming healthy fiber from vegetables, fruits, grains, and beans will assist the intestines for more regular elimination.

On average, women require twenty to twenty-five grams of fiber each day, and men thirty to thirty-eight grams daily for smooth elimination in that department.

The more waste we remove, the better the body becomes at removing it, and the healthier you will be.

And don't forget to flush! It's a courtesy, after all.

CHAPTER 18
BRAIN HEALTH

When health is absent, wisdom cannot reveal itself, art
cannot manifest, strength cannot fight, wealth becomes
useless, and intelligence cannot be applied.

—Herophilus

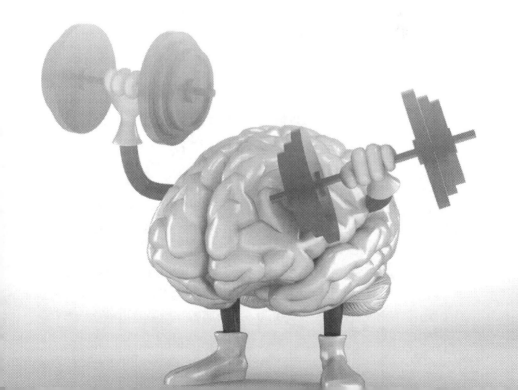

When I was fifty-one years old, I had attempted nearly every physical and mental challenge I could handle and pushed myself to the limits.

You may have guessed the next obvious step: taking private hip-hop lessons. I wasn't a bad dancer, often dancing around my home. I had even won a dance contest years back. My Boy-band fantasies are long gone, but perhaps Old Kids on the Block shouldn't be ruled out.

I called the LA Dancefit studio in West Los Angeles and set up a lesson with the owner, Wil. Dance is as natural to Wil as health is to me, and we immediately became good friends.

After two lessons, Wil asked if I wanted to participate in the spring group performance. Sure, why not? The lessons felt incredible, so why not take them to the next level of performance.

I was nervous. To try and be a part of a troop of seasoned hip-hop enthusiasts would be a challenge, and I'd have to prove my worth and keep up and not make them look bad or have to leave.

I anxiously walked into the first rehearsal. There were twenty-seven people; I was the only male. The group of women aged from twenty to seventy-one; none had ever performed a hip-hop routine solo or in a troop. Holy S! We were going to be the Bad News Bears of hip-hop troops.

Wil had a three-and-a-half-minute routine for us to perform choreographed to the Bruno Mars hit song "Perm."

I remained optimistic we could pull it off, and happy I did.

After the first of the eight rehearsals, a performance seemed impossible. But by our eighth, we actually felt like a troop. We were not ready for World of Dance, but I felt we at least would make it through the routine.

The twenty-eight of us took to the stage in our funky matching galactic space-themed sweatsuits and gold mirror-finished shoes with blinking LED lights in the soles and thoroughly funked it up for the 350 people watching in the Santa Monica Middle School auditorium.

Those eight weeks stimulated my brain in many ways; I began to paint again and refocused my creativity on fitness choreography. Thank you again, Wil, for such an enjoyable and impactful experience.

NEUROPLASTICITY

The brain needs external challenges to stimulate neuroplasticity: the brain's ability to form new neurons from adapting to your physical environment and mental demands.

As important as physical exercise is for muscles, neuroplasticity is crucial for sustaining brain health and mitigating the loss of cognitive function as we age. A loss of neuroplasticity can increase the likelihood of neurodegenerative illnesses like Alzheimer's and Parkinson's.

When the body is inactive; or only moves in the same simple patterns, needed health-providing neurological and brain-developing requests are absent.

Make neuroplasticity a regular practice for helping you to maintain optimal brain and body health.

SIMPLE WAYS TO STIMULATE NEUROPLASTICITY

- Choose a different route to work or school.
- Learn an instrument.
- Take a dance or martial arts class.
- Research a challenging new subject.
- Begin learning a new language.
- Brush the teeth or eat with your non-dominant hand.
- Alternate standing on one leg instead of both while online or idly waiting.
- Throw a ping-pong ball against a barrier or wall to improve hand-to-eye coordination while at the same time stimulating neuroplasticity.

PROPRIOCEPTION

Proprioception is the brain's ability to perceive the body's position and location in space. Proprioception is present in every movement we make.

Proprioception is brain training in three dimensions. The better your proprioceptive abilities, the better our kinesthetic body awareness becomes.

Any balance exercises or movement over any terrain or obstacles benefits proprioception and the brain's ability to connect to the body and be aware of your relation to your surroundings.

PROPRIOCEPTION MOVES

- Standing on one leg.
- Side leg lifts and rear leg lifts
- Forward or reverse lunge
- Walking a straight line as if on a balance beam
- Hiking or walking uneven terrain

Close your eyes during safe movements in controlled atmospheres to intensify the neuromuscular effects.

THE POWER OF THE PARIETAL LOBE

In addition to physical movements, reading further stimulates the brain for development.

Reading engages the parietal lobe, which turns letters you see into words and the words read into thoughts and promotes imagination, creativity, memory retention, and decision-making abilities.

Entertaining as they are, viewing movies and television does not produce the equivalent parietal effect on the brain as reading provides.

CHAPTER 19

PROCREATION IS OUR PURPOSE

You were designed for accomplishment, engineered for success, and endowed with the seeds of greatness.

—Zig Ziglar

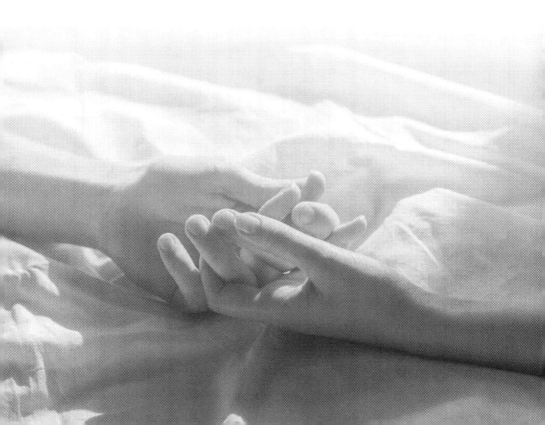

PRIMAL INSTINCTS HARD-WIRED IN OUR DNA

- The need for food
- Procreating (sex)
- Protecting ourselves from danger

SEXUAL HEALTH AND HORMONES

The hormones estrogen and testosterone are responsible for keeping the body feeling good and looking young.

Estrogen stimulates younger-looking skin, beautifies hair and nails, and regulates the menstrual cycle, reproductive tract, urinary tract, heart, blood vessels, bone health, breasts, mucous membranes, pelvic muscles, and the brain.

Testosterone, often thought of as the male hormone also plays a big part in women's health. For women, testosterone is essential for bone and breast health, fertility, menstrual regularity, and vaginal health.

In men, testosterone levels affect body fat distribution, bone density, facial and body hair, mood, muscle growth, strength, production of sperm, and sex drive.

Regular sexual activity helps boost the production of these hormones to naturally build immunity to better defend against bacteria, viruses, germs, and common illnesses.

CLIMACTIC RESULTS

Orgasms improve circulation throughout the entire body; and release endorphins and the hormone oxytocin, which reduces pain, and stress; while elevating mood state.

PROSTATE AND HEART
HEALTH FOR MEN

Men should practice a balanced diet, get sun or use vitamin D supplements, and ejaculate regularly to help sleep, improve sperm quality, boost the immune system, and reduce the risk of heart disease and prostate cancer.

CONNECT

When we are sexually active, it signals our nervous system for vitality; and drives us to feel more energized, young, and connected.

Being sexually active is also an obvious opportunity to bond, receive love, and give affection. Never disregard or ignore the influence of sexual health; embrace and look forward to it. Maintaining sexual health is as important as consistently balanced nutrition.

CHAPTER 20

HEALTH TECHNOLOGIES THAT MAKE A DIFFERENCE

Technology is a gift of God. After the gift of life, it is
perhaps the greatest of God's gifts. It is the mother
of civilizations, of arts, and of sciences.

—Freeman Dyson

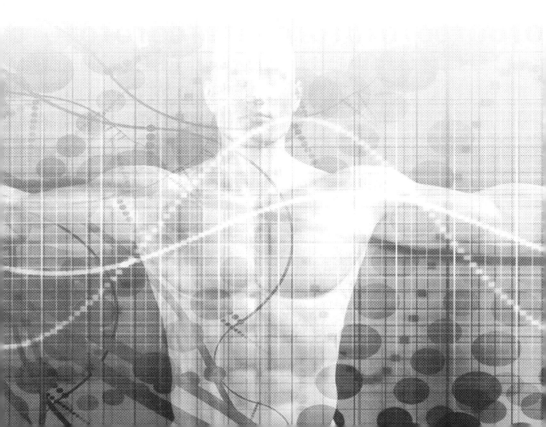

Through the years of continued research and application, I have found numerous irreplaceable non-invasive modalities that I use daily to give me a metabolic edge without ever over-taxing my body.

For years, daily, I have utilized these three healing modalities to enhance my health, heal and recover with more years to come.

- Red light therapy
- Bemer therapy
- Vibration training

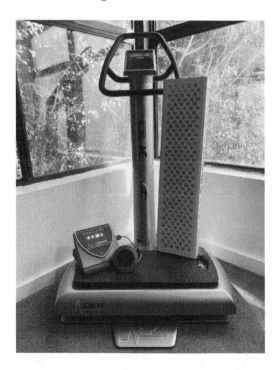

If you do not like to exert yourself, you will enjoy these life-enhancing health technologies that create health benefits while you lay, sit, or remain stationary to use them. They were all developed to improve circulation, increase blood oxygenation, stimulate waste removal, and build cellular integrity without you having to break a sweat.

RED LIGHT THERAPY

Light exists in a broad spectrum of wavelengths that we need to absorb for optimal health.

Red light and infrared light fall within the wavelength range of 620–750 nm and benefit the function of our cells significantly.

Red light therapy devices deliver specific wavelengths that stimulate the sense of well-being that we experience after spending time outdoors in the sun, without the dangerous UVA and UVB wavelengths that cause premature aging and skin cancer.

Red light within this range penetrates deep into the skin, offering visible rejuvenating effects that can help resolve a wide range of health conditions. Our cells absorb red light and infrared light and convert this into energy to build new proteins, collagen, and elastin, and improve cellular regeneration.

Red-light therapy helps the body absorb vitamin D for maintaining health when going outdoors is not an option and is safe and just as effective for your pets and plants.

NEAR-INFRARED THERAPY

Visible red light is only half of the light therapy spectrum; near-infrared light (NIR) is the second half.

NIR is above the visible light spectrum with wavelengths ranging from 700 nm to over 1,100 nm.

NIR wavelengths of 800–880 offer exceptional therapeutic benefits of healing and cellular regeneration.

The body absorbs NIR light in our cells the same way as visible red light.

NIR wavelengths are longer and penetrate deeper into body tissue than visible red light.

Red light wavelengths penetrate the skin, promoting collagen production and skin clarity. NIR light can penetrate much deeper into the body's tissue to target deep wounds, injuries, sore muscles, and joint pain.

Red-light and NIR therapy can reach into the cell's mitochondria, helping improve appearance, physical performance, and overall well-being.

My Usage: Twenty minutes a day, four to six days a week, always with a glass of water.

BEMER THERAPY

There are two primary energy sources: light energy waves and sound energy waves. Red light and Near-Infrared Red therapy; use light wave energy, while Bemer therapy utilizes inaudible sound waves to increase circulation and reduce inflammation throughout the vast capillary network throughout the body to promote healing and improved health.

The BEMER name stands for bioelectric magnetic energy regulation. BEMER helps improve the blood flow to the smallest vessels of the circulatory system.

Bemer improves the delivery of nutrients to the body's cells while helping eliminate metabolic waste and increasing oxygen levels in the blood by nearly 30%.

BEMER therapy can improve every one's life and help people suffering from chronic conditions, musculo-skeletal pain, fatigue, peripheral vascular disease, migraines, vertigo, and chronic health conditions related to reduced blood flow.

World-class athletes and trainers use Bemer therapy to improve physical performance, shorten recovery time, and rehabilitate from injuries.

BEMER is an exceptional healing tool; in addition to my daily use. In 2019 I was hit by a car that crushed a joint in my left fifth metatarsal and fractured my left ankle. I committed to BEMER therapy multiple times a day following the accident. The added circulation healed my injuries seven weeks sooner than the doctor's original diagnosis.

My Usage: Daily use of eight minutes in the morning and eight minutes at night. When I need to recover from injuries, I use Bemer several hours each day to accelerate healing.

VIBRATION TRAINING

Whole Body Vibration uses precise mechanical oscillations to create therapeutic muscular contractions known as involuntary neuromuscular stretch reflex reactions.

Vibration training frequency ranges from 25 Hz–to 50 Hz per second, moving in a cyclical two to four-millimeter vertical motion that increases blood flow, balance, joint strength, bone density, flexibility, proprioceptive sense, and endurance.

Vibration training can also reduce the symptoms associated with restless leg syndrome without the need for medication.

My Usage: Two minutes each morning at 45 hz–50 hz and two minutes at 40 hz–45 hz before sleep.

CHAPTER 21

ENERGY EXCHANGE

If only you could sense how important you are to the lives of
those you meet; how important you can be to people you
may never even dream of. There is something of yourself
that you leave at every meeting with another person.

—Fred Rogers

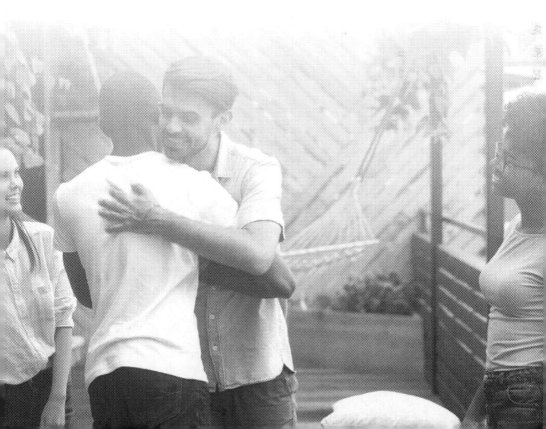

I was returning to the dorm when I was a freshman at the University of Southern California; in the fall of 1985; and walking through the second-floor hallway of Flour Tower when I noticed a girl crouched on the floor, obviously crying; and nobody was paying attention. I stopped to ask, "Are you okay?"

"No, I'm not," she replied

"Okay, do you need some help?"

"Only if you can dance!"

I didn't quite understand that. "What do you mean?"

"I have tickets to be a dancer on Dick Clark's nighttime TV show, but my friends think it's stupid, and I've asked everyone, and it's tonight, and no one will go, and I hate this place."

"Ok, I'll go with you," I said.

She paused, looked at me inquisitively, and said, "Can you even dance?"

I nodded and did a 360 spin, ending with an open arm finish and a smile.

"We leave in forty-five minutes!" she said, then popped up and ran down the hall.

"Ah, what's your name? I'm Michael, Carson!" I said loud enough for her to hear while running away.

"Great, I'm Dana; meet me at the front door in forty-five minutes—no, forty! Don't be late, Michael Carson!"

"OK, nice to mee—" She was gone!

Nighttime was the evening version of Dick Clark's *American Bandstand*. The audience danced to Top 40 hits and pop band performances. It was my first time on a TV production. We recorded eight shows in two days.

The show also held a dance contest every fourth show. The judges chose competitors from the audience, and they chose us; and three other couples.

We were so excited; we were going to compete for a prize on national television. We rehearsed a few moves while the production set the stage and waited eagerly to hear the song choice for the competition. The 80s had hundreds of great dance hits; it could be a Madonna song, Prince, Stevie Wonder, or maybe Janet Jackson? We could tear up the floor with any of those songs.

But, the Nighttime staff chose a Dire Straits tune, "Walk of Life." It had to look funny on camera because all the couples needed to take a beat to absorb what we were listening to before anybody could begin to dance. It was not the perfect song, but we were determined. Our moves resembled a combination of the diner dance scene from Pulp Fiction and Riverdance. Not our most graceful moment.

When the song ended, we were all wiped out and gasping for breath while Mr. Clark assigned us team numbers, asked us our names, and showed us the Casio CT810 piano synthesizers one couple would be winning. Then Mr. Clark said, "Judge, you have been watching in the control room, oh, electronic dancing voice of doom, and the winner is couple number...?"

We hear through the intercom, "Number three!"

We were number three. We won! Oh my god! Now I had to learn how to play the keyboard. What a fun experience.

When we were back at the dorm, if I had responded like the rest of the people, both Dana and I would have missed out on an experience to cherish. Life-changing moments are everywhere; the only limitation is not to recognize them.

Humans have an instinctual need to be acknowledged, to belong, be accepted, and feel included by our fellow humans. Have you ever experienced the uneasy feeling when approaching a stranger, sharing an elevator, or waiting in line?

On the occasions when a person or people made attempts to say hello, or you made an effort to greet someone, that uneasy feeling most likely disappeared.

Uneasy feelings can remain until you make a connection or the circumstance passes.

Recognition from others directly impacts psychological and physical health, subconscious effects on breathing, blood flow, posture, and self-worth. Being disregarded by our fellow humans can cause feelings of rejection, isolation, or anxiety.

It's healthy, necessary, and human nature for people to acknowledge each other. A connection elevates the mood states of everyone, increases social skills, and improves self-esteem.

Make an effort to connect with your fellow humans, embrace a potential opportunity to learn, share ideas, and experience the positive energy created when two or more people form a genuine connection.

You are a powerful energy source; the more you connect, the more you build collective power for all of us. Singularly, we burn like candles, and collectively we roar like a bonfire.

CHAPTER 22

THE RELATIONSHIP BETWEEN THE CONSCIOUS AND SUBCONSCIOUS

When you recover or discover something that nourishes your soul and brings joy, care enough about yourself to make room for it in your life.

—Jean Shinoda Bolen

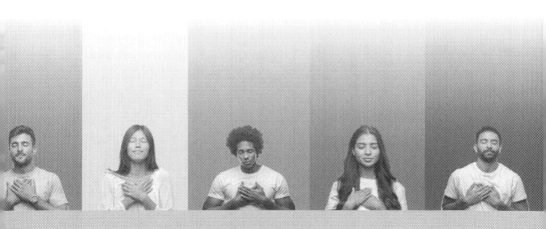

I recommend reading or listening to the influential book Feeling is the Secret by Neville Goddard, first introduced to me by my dear friend Shahin. Goodard shares the role our subconscious plays in determining our conscious reality; and provides strategies to help you realize your desires to enable powerful improvements in your conscious world.

When we prepare to sleep each night and leave the waking conscious world, we have no choice but to bring our last thoughts and emotions into our subconscious sleep state and agree with them as being fact. It is a human characteristic we all share and cannot avoid. The subconscious eagerly accepts these emotions.

In the book, Neville shares specific practices to enhance the relationship between the subconscious and conscious to help you better attain your goals through sleep, meditation, and intention.

The book will take you roughly an hour to read, and has the potential to change the rest of your life.

CHAPTER 23
GRATITUDE

Fall in love with becoming the best version of yourself, but with patience, with compassion and respect to your own journey.

—S. McNutt

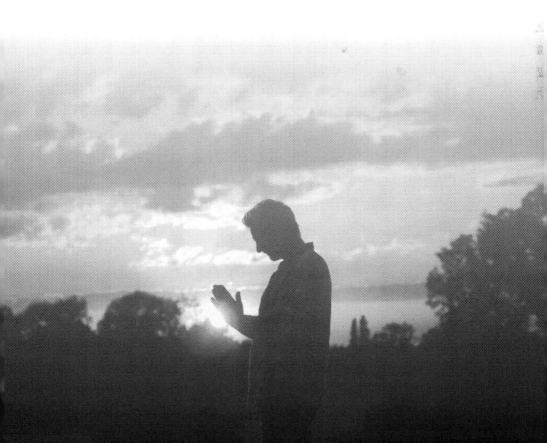

My ally, health, continues to furnish me with the energy of my youth. The lifestyle adaptations I make throughout my health journey will continue to evolve and improve as I learn more about myself, my health, and how to increase longevity. Thankfulness and appreciation are potent ways I tap into immediately improving my mood state and nurturing my mental health.

I make an effort to focus on exceptional thoughts and look beyond the unfavorable. Gratitude will build with practice. You can create appreciation and feel the emotional benefits anytime; and anyplace.

Gratitude builds a positive redirection of thought and leads to increased optimism. Studies show that optimism and positive thoughts elevate emotions, heighten circulation, and help maintain heart health.

Negative thoughts and anger; can restrict circulation and lead to fear, anxiety, and depression. Gratitude is a powerful tool for shining bright light into any darkness. When in a state of gratitude, negative emotions are squelched and replaced with positive ones. It is not possible to have negative thoughts while practicing gratitude.

Experiencing gratitude releases the hormone dopamine, eliciting positive emotions, optimism, and camaraderie.

Take time for moments of gratitude as often as you remember. Include four to six breaths to reflect, reboot, and naturally alleviate tension and negative emotions.

I hope the concepts and strategies I shared with you help enlighten and simplify your path to personal health. Thank you from the bottom of my very healthy heart; for joining me on our ongoing health journey.

With gratitude,
Michael & Freeway

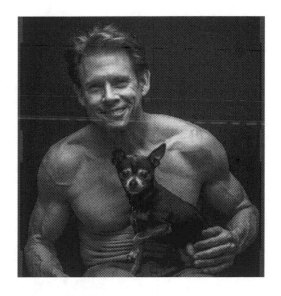

QUICK HEALTHY TIPS

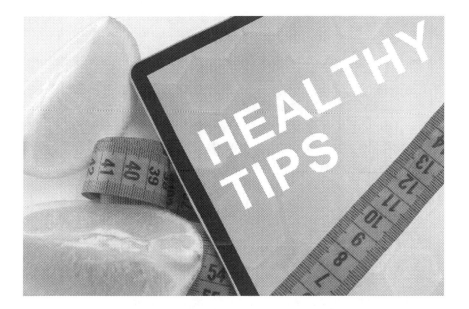

1. SITTING TOO LONG

- You can relieve the body from sitting too long by stimulating circulation to the glutes, lower back, and hips.
- Begin by sitting tall, feet flat on the floor, engage the glutes by squeezing them tightly together while pressing firmly down through the feet.
- Hold the glute contraction for one to two seconds while exhaling. Release and repeat for fifteen to twenty reps.

- Rest thirty seconds, then perform a second round of glute squeezes. Remember to exhale when contracting the muscles.
- Then from sitting to standing, perform fifteen to twenty squats from a seated position after completing the second set of glute squeezes. Reach upward with your arms as you rise from the squats. Squeeze the glutes for one second at the top of each rep.

This simple routine can provide a tremendous amount of relief from sitting while also building the muscles in these areas to support you better.

2. THE POWER OF A SMILE

- When answering the phone, make an effort to smile when saying hello and talking.
- Always smile when greeting someone. There is no better feeling than receiving a warm welcome, and a smile will set the tone for the experience. Notice how conversations elevate to new levels.
- For a quick mental reset, smile for ten to fifteen seconds while thinking of your desires and allow the warm feeling to sink in.

3. RECOVERY FROM INJURIES

- When recovering from an injury or surgery, consume more vegetables and less bread and pasta; to naturally keep inflammation down and a more expedited recovery.

4. ALWAYS BE PREPARED TO MOVE

- Keep a pair of running or walking shoes in the car or luggage when traveling, and go for a walk when time allows. There is no pressure to run; walking will clear the head, and the cross-crawl activity will produce better clarity in your brain.
- After long drives, flights, or when seated for an extended time, take a quick walk to reset the body; and as a natural way to boost energy.
- Go outside for walks in the daytime sun when traveling to help quickly reset your internal clock for the local time zone.

5. BURN EXTRA CALORIES

- Park farther from the entrance when going to the store or running errands.
- Take the stairs when able.
- When rising from a chair, perform a few squats that warm up the legs and body and you will even continue to burn more calories for several

minutes to follow. These small steps add up to significant results.

6. ALKALINE WITH EASE

- Squeezing a fresh lemon wedge into drinking water helps to alkalize your system and aids in the digestion of food. It also provides a dose of vitamin C, boosts potassium, and tastes great. Cut a lemon into six to eight wedges and get six to eight glasses of alkaline per lemon.

7. HIDE THE SCALE AND REMOVE ANXIETY

- Hide the scale, store it, throw it away, donate it, or at least avoid it. The number revealed is never going to be as important as how you feel.

8. WARM-UP FIRST, STRETCH SECOND

- Stretching muscles when cold and stiff; can cause a strain, sprain, or even tearing. A simple five to seven-minute warm-up provides muscles and tendons needed circulation and increased heat to allow the muscles to stretch more freely, lessening the chance of injuries.

9. MUSIC ELEVATES YOUR MOOD

- Music has the power to ultimately elevate our moods. The more music there is in your life, the happier you will be.
- Play music you enjoy and dance, play air guitar or drums, and just let go of tension.

10. WHEN FEELING DOWN, DEPRESSED, OR LOST

- No matter our life experiences, finding gratitude in even the most minor things will cause a mental shift into positivity that affects mental and physical chemistry. We are blessed even in the worst of times. Recognizing this is a powerful tool. I have included gratitude a second time due to its remarkable power of positivity.

Printed in the United States
by Baker & Taylor Publisher Services